BROKEN MIND, PERSISTENT HOPE

BROKEN MIND, PERSISTENT HOPE

A Memoir of Recovery from
Brain Damage and Manic Depression

Thomas E. Hartmann

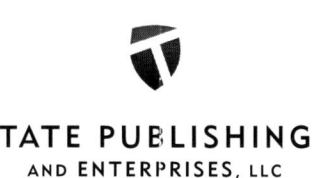

TATE PUBLISHING
AND ENTERPRISES, LLC

Broken Mind, Persistent Hope
Copyright © 2014 by Thomas E. Hartmann. All rights reserved.

No part of this publication may be reproduced, stored in a retrieval system or transmitted in any way by any means, electronic, mechanical, photocopy, recording or otherwise without the prior permission of the author except as provided by USA copyright law.

The opinions expressed by the author are not necessarily those of Tate Publishing, LLC.

Published by Tate Publishing & Enterprises, LLC
127 E. Trade Center Terrace | Mustang, Oklahoma 73064 USA
1.888.361.9473 | www.tatepublishing.com

Tate Publishing is committed to excellence in the publishing industry. The company reflects the philosophy established by the founders, based on Psalm 68:11,

"The Lord gave the word and great was the company of those who published it."

Book design copyright © 2014 by Tate Publishing, LLC. All rights reserved.

Published in the United States of America

ISBN: 978-1-62902-148-5
1. Biography & Autobiography / Personal Memoirs
2. Psychology / Mental Illness
14.09.19

"Educate the patient, medical journals advise clinicians, and [thus] solve the problems of non-compliance that plague the treatment of chronic disease."

—Byron J. Good, "Medical Anthropology and the Problem of Belief,"
in *Medicine, Rationality, and Experience*

"Feeling slightly silly, I dared to pronounce the words only silently, inside my head: 'I ask the Healer inside me to come out and heal this woman.'"

—Olga Kharitidi, *Entering the Circle: Ancient Secrets of Siberian Wisdom Discovered by a Russian Psychiatrist*

Contents

Part I Confused Kid

Chapter 1	Old Rag	3
Chapter 2	Mama Mia	5
Chapter 3	In Nazi Germany	11
Chapter 4	Naughty Boy	15
Chapter 5	Just Desserts	19
Chapter 6	Dad Hosts the Mongol Horde	21
Chapter 7	Saved by the Computer	25
Chapter 8	First Love	31
Chapter 9	Heady Perestroika	37
Chapter 10	To Russia With Love	41
Chapter 11	Cycling for Peace With the KGB	45
Chapter 12	Bottoms Up	51
Chapter 13	Marriage Without Mom	57

Part II Into the Abyss

Chapter 14	The Real World	63
Chapter 15	*Deutschland*	67
Chapter 16	Over the Edge	71
Chapter 17	Fairy Tales	75
Chapter 18	Shock Therapy	79
Chapter 19	*Nyet!*	85
Chapter 20	*Desantnik*	89
Chapter 21	Homeward	97

Chapter 22	The Pear Cure	103
Chapter 23	"What Seems to Be the Problem?"	107
Chapter 24	Flipping Eggs	111
Chapter 25	Back for Seconds	115
Chapter 26	Tatiana's Turn	121
Chapter 27	T-Boned by an Eighteen-Wheeler	125

Part III Smothered by Diagnoses

Chapter 28	Two Times Lucky	131
Chapter 29	Looking in on Me	135
Chapter 30	Withdrawal Pangs	141
Chapter 31	Dr. Schwein	145
Chapter 32	Humbled	151
Chapter 33	Just Being Friendly	157
Chapter 34	Locked Up Again	161
Chapter 35	Inmates	167
Chapter 36	Tatiana's Visit	173
Chapter 37	Isolation	179
Chapter 38	Paradigm Shift	183

Part IV Treatment at Home

Chapter 39	"Learn a Language"	191
Chapter 40	Shanghaied	195
Chapter 41	Monkey Mind	201
Chapter 42	Salt for Sale	205
Chapter 43	Calling the Professor	209

Chapter 44	Smiley Faces	213
Chapter 45	Think Fast	217
Chapter 46	Rain	221
Chapter 47	Pills From Tibet	225
Chapter 48	M&M's at the Orchestra	231
Chapter 49	Shamanic Healing	235
Chapter 50	Descent Into Madness	239

Part V On My Own

Chapter 51	The Cuckoo's Nest Again	245
Chapter 52	"I Am the Idiot"	251
Chapter 53	Busted	257
Chapter 54	Farewell	265
Chapter 55	Stretched Too Far	277
Chapter 56	First Date	283
Chapter 57	How to Make a Good Impression	289
Chapter 58	Finding Home	293
Chapter 59	A Second Chance	301
Chapter 60	Thank God I Married a Saint	305
Chapter 61	Climbing Mount Sinai	309
Epilogue		317
Chronology		318

Those with brain damage and mental illness are people, too. This fact can sometimes be overlooked by those who see few prospects for recovery. I hope my return to sanity and normal functioning will inspire both patients and doctors to see beyond the limitations of contemporary medicine and envision a day when these afflictions will be as treatable as a broken bone.

Some names have been changed in the following account to protect the privacy of family and friends. Otherwise all events related are true to the best of my memory.

T.E.H.
Havertown, Pennsylvania
2013

PART I

CONFUSED KID

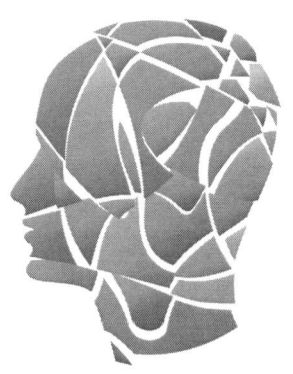

CHAPTER 1

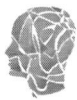

Old Rag

Diane, some thirty years my senior, was hiking with me up Old Rag, one of the summits in New York's Adirondack Mountains. We were just reaching the tree line, where evergreens gave way to sheer rock. I was only twelve. Diane was my mother's lover and shared her passion for hiking. My mother was heading up the trail a few minutes behind us.

With youthful enthusiasm I scrambled up the rockface in front of us, wanting to be the first to the top. My sturdy hiking boots grabbed the gray stone. By holding on to the mountain with my short arms I made faster progress than Diane could ever hope for. Soon I was alone.

Wind began to pick up near the top. I leaned into it, catching sight of the breathtaking vista. Clouds covered some of the valleys and rounded green mountains rose between them. This view was what we had come for. Elated, I scampered over the rock, not really looking where I was going. Suddenly I found myself on the ground with a scrape on my right arm. Yikes! I was bleeding. What if my mom and Diane never found me?

I began to panic. "Mom! Diane! Help!" I scrambled back in their direction. Diane, of course, was right behind me, but by that point I was in a frenzy.

"Tom, it's okay. It's okay."

"Where's Mom? I hurt myself! Look!"

"Tom, it's okay. She'll be right here. It's okay."

I was not comforted. Her words only served to heighten my panic. I wanted my mommy and Diane was just a friend.

I had hit my funny bone in the fall. "It hurts! O-o-o-o-ow! A-a-a-ah . . ."

I was in the middle of a wail when Diane slapped me across my left cheek. "Get a grip on yourself, Tom."

I shut my mouth and looked up at her, astonished. Just then my mother appeared out of the trees below. She summed up the situation in a glance. Maybe she had even overheard our interaction.

"Did you just hit Tom?" she asked calmly, slowing her pace to join us. She had not seen the violence but sensed it in my expression.

"He was completely out of control," Diane said.

"If I you ever hit him again, Diane," my mother said evenly, "it's over between us." She took off her pack and pulled out a small red first aid kit. I gasped with relief at her touch.

CHAPTER 2

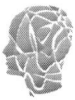

Mama Mia

Nine years later, I lay on a couch in my father's living room, my mouth pounding from the recent removal of wisdom teeth. But my heart was on wings: I was in love. I had recently returned from a summer in Germany, where I had studied the language during the day and pursued one of the first women I met with tender devotion. I was twenty-one. She was big hearted, in fact a little overweight, and we had put off consummating our romance until my final evening in the country. In my pain, I thought only of her.

Then steps marched across the porch, rousing me from my reverie. Some paper shuffled, the mail slot clicked, and the steps faded away. What could this be? Our mail had already arrived. I scrambled to my feet and investigated the mystery. Perhaps my love had sent a telegram?

On the letter was scrawled "To Tom." The handwriting was distinctively my mother's. I tore it open. "I cannot deal with you anymore," it began. "I am divorcing you."

I felt the rug being pulled out from under me. Her support of me, once so powerful, had receded as I established my identity in adolescence. At first I couldn't accept her words, but then slowly I realized that she was capable of this.

I remembered the bitter and caustic divorce she had initiated with my father fifteen years earlier, before Diane had ever come on the scene. She had sued for the house and, when she didn't win, settled into an apartment, happy to support herself as a microscopy expert at nearby DuPont, a job my father had arranged for her in lieu of alimony.

She had no desire for custody of me and my sister in her apartment. At the time we were aged six and seven, respectively. We were left behind with her husband and the house. She even refused to talk to any of us for months after the divorce.

When the better part of a year had passed, she offered to take us out for fast food over the weekends. She also invited us along for her vacations. Could a mother really divorce her son? If anyone could, it was Ingeborg.

My teeth now really began to hurt, and tears welled up. "What's the matter, Thomas?" my father asked, having just come up from the basement. I thrust the letter into his hands and threw myself onto the couch, holding my shaking head.

"Oh, Tomchen . . ." my father said gently, using the affectionate German name he had used with me as a child. He sat down next to me and put his arm around my shoulder. "Give her time. She's just in a bad mood."

As a toddler I had basked in my mother's attention. She had made every attempt to train me to be a child prodigy, and I had risen to the challenge. Back then it had been easy for me to please her and our relationship had made me feel safe and loved, but as her marriage soured, so did she, and of course I took it personally. I never recovered from the divorce and the feeling of rejection that came when she left. As soon as she was out of the house, she began her six-month "sabbatical from motherhood," cutting off all contact with us while she reestablished herself. I felt abandoned.

Just over a year before that, prior to our move to Wilmington, she had suffered a small stroke. It left her a different woman, but not in a way apparent to others: she became aware of her mortality. It seemed that she feared the limitations that could result from a stroke and, at thirty-five, made a firm decision to maintain control of her life by killing herself when she reached seventy. Whether to psyche herself up for it or to remind her loved ones to appreciate her while they had her, she affirmed her planned suicide to us regularly.

Ever since I was five, I had been hearing how she was going to make her "final exit" in the foreseeable future. I had developed considerable anxiety about the possibility of losing her, so even as a man of twenty-one I was devastated when she "divorced" me.

I decided to call her bluff and take her to a see a shrink. Psychologists set crazy people straight, and any woman who wants to divorce her son is crazy by definition. I thought I could outsmart her, but Ingeborg was easy to underestimate.

When I called later, her very measured "okay" made me wonder if something was fishy. "Sure, let's go to a therapist. Only I choose. And I pay." She had me there: of course it would cost money. I hadn't even thought of that. Then the line clicked dead.

My father, in the meantime, was cooking. I sat in my usual spot at the kitchen table. "What's for dinner?" I asked.

"How about peeling some potatoes, Thomas?"

"Dad, I'm sorry, I don't really feel like it. My teeth hurt. How could Mom be that mean?" I said.

"She's just not functioning very well as a mother."

My father took the potatoes from the fridge himself and began peeling them. Just then the telephone rang. I hopped up and took notes.

"Okay, five-thirty. The office is across from the restaurant." I wrote down the doctor's name. Again the phone clicked.

"Save some dinner for me, Dad. I'm sure a doctor can figure this out. Can I borrow your car?"

He nodded, concentrating on the food. I grabbed the keys and ran out.

A light rain was falling when I turned off Concord Pike into the parking lot. My mother stood in front of one of the entrances, glancing at her watch. "You're two minutes late."

"Sorry, Mom." When I was in tenth grade, she had asked me to call her by her first name, Ingeborg. Not only did I hate the sound of "Ingeborg," but out of a certain longing for intimacy I had never followed through on her request.

This was my first visit to a psychologist. As we ascended the narrow stairs to the office, I felt slightly uneasy. My mother seemed so sure of what she was doing.

It felt stuffy sitting there with her in front of *Time* and *Good Housekeeping* magazines and a closed door, neither of us speaking to the other. Suddenly a forty-something woman emerged and smiled at us. "Ingeborg and Thomas Hartmann?" she asked. "Which of you would like to come in first?"

Before I could even think to answer, my mother volunteered and I was alone. Why the haste? Well, not to worry . . . surely the doctor would solve this problem. I glanced through articles, trying to put myself at ease.

I had finished *Time* magazine and was starting in on *Good Housekeeping* when the door finally opened. Caught off guard by the therapist's chumminess with my mom, I suddenly realized that I was out in the cold. "Mr. Hartmann?" the doctor said, smiling.

My mother and I passed each other without exchanging glances. The therapist closed the door behind me. "So," I mustered, sitting across from her in a chair. "What do you make of all this?"

The doctor looked me straight in the eye. "She doesn't want to be your mother anymore. She says you're inconsiderate, and that you didn't bring her a gift when you came back from Germany."

Her finality caught me off guard. Was that it? She regarded me calmly as her words sank in. All of a sudden I realized that Ingeborg was probably leaving without me and involuntarily jumped from my seat, wondering what I was doing in that sterile office. Longing for my mother, I excused myself, burst through two office doors, and skipped down the steps to see if I could catch her before I was alone.

Ingeborg's car was idling in the pouring rain, headlights on. As she pulled away, I ran up to her driver's side door. "You can't do this!" I yelled. She rolled down her window.

"Watch me," she said as she rolled it back up and eased out of the parking spot.

CHAPTER 3

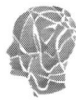

In Nazi Germany

As my mother drove away, I could feel my heart tightening. I figured I would give her a dose of her own medicine. I resolved to shut her out. I would prove that I could get by just fine without her. After all, I was an adult, already out of school. I affirmed to myself that I would thrive, even without a sense of my mother's love. It didn't occur to me then that closing my heart might leave lasting scars on it.

Who knows how many unhappy generations there had been in Ingeborg's family? Her father, the story goes, as a child had spent a year responding to all questions with only "Yes," "No," or "Maybe." A year! Later, when I tried to trace insanity in the family, he became a prime suspect. Back in his small German town, complete with a castle by the river, he had owned the factory where just about everyone worked. On Sundays his elegant family, including the young Ingeborg, would take a stroll and nod to the townspeople.

"Anyone in the family who asked where we were headed had to stay home," she would often say later, to give us a taste of her childhood.

As soon as she was a young adult, Ingeborg got out of that town, I suspect with a warped soul. She spent a few years in Stuttgart studying electron microscopy, then resolved to come to America to settle. She moved to Cambridge, Massachusetts, and dated German Fulbright scholars, but she couldn't find anyone who wanted to stay.

As she described it, eventually there was only my father left, an East German immigrant who by no means wanted to go back. They married almost by default. Four years later, I was born, a year after my sister Julia.

"I never wanted a second child, especially not a boy. I cursed you *in utero*." She often showed a streak of honesty that left me feeling as unwelcome as I probably was. Sometimes she would soften it with, "I only fell in love with you once you were born."

Our family eventually settled in a three-story brick house in Wilmington, Delaware. Ingeborg, never comfortable with motherhood, had approached it as something of an academic discipline. The truth is that she was hankering for a job in science. She never wanted to come to Wilmington because it meant leaving behind a career opportunity that had presented itself in her narrow field just before the move.

We kids began to hear more and more arguments between our parents. It turned out that Ingeborg had started planning for a divorce soon after we arrived in Delaware. The two of them camped out in separate bedrooms. The emerging women's movement caught her fancy and served her purposes, but she took it to unrealistic extremes.

Getting a refugee father out of his American home was too much of a challenge, even for Ingeborg and her lawyers. As she marched down the stairs, armed with suitcases, I was beside myself. "Mommy! Don't go! Pl-e-e-e-ease!" I followed her out to her orange VW bug, but she was unmoved.

After Ingeborg moved out, however, something in me shifted. Once a tidy kid, I turned into a complete slob. And I began to steal at school.

CHAPTER 4

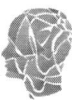

Naughty Boy

I thought the shelf of my own locker—wasn't that supposed to be private?—would make a good hiding place for the shiny rubber ball I had swiped from the governor's son. But at my private school, where Delaware's elite were educated, lockers had no locks. I thought I had gotten away with it when our class sat in a circle, and I responded with silence when our teacher asked, "Does anyone know what happened to the shiny ball?"

* * *

"Well, Thomas, the bad news is that starting next week you will be going to public school. The good news is that you will be skipping a grade." My father had just met with the principal. He looked as if he'd been put through a shredder.

I was confused. "Julia, too?"

"No, just you, I'm afraid. This divorce has taken its toll on all of us and we can't afford to send you to private school anymore, just Julia." My jaw dropped. "Ingeborg will be paying tuition for her out of the money she gets from that job I arranged as part of the settlement, but I'm afraid there's no way I'm going to be able to pay for you."

Close to forty years passed before I realized that I had been expelled from school over the theft of my influential friend's ball. Trying to make sense out of it at the time, I concluded that, true to her allusions to never wanting a son, my mother had actually never valued me the way she valued my sister and that my father didn't think I was worth the cost of school. Either that or he was too much of a cheapskate to foot the bill. That would jibe with what Ingeborg had been saying about him all along.

Perhaps the divorce would have gone more smoothly if Ingeborg had not resented my father so much. Her attitude toward our father translated into bitterness toward all of us. During the period that she was signed off from motherhood she even hung up on us when we called, giving us a silent treatment reminiscent of her father back in Germany. My dad dealt with our inevitable sniffles and scraped knees, but only with the help of a sympathetic pediatrician. "I can't believe she is doing this to her own children," I remember the doctor saying as she administered my immunizations.

Ingeborg never really enjoyed cooking. For meals, she often ate dried milk powder. Her stove burners heated water, but, reflecting her own priorities, she converted the oven to hardware storage and let the broiler serve as a toolbox. That setup actually made sense in her limited living space, but to a child who longed for cuddling and tender care, it had a hard edge.

She packed Julia and me into her car after dinner at our father's place on Fridays. Then we would spend Saturdays with her, often taking trips to the countryside where her lover Diane lived. When we were with her alone, we often ate at McDonald's.

"Your father is so cheap—really second class. You can't believe him when he talks," she told us with conviction. I was all ears. After all, didn't that explain why I was in public school? "He's a politician, but I tell it like it is."

She sure did tell it like it was. Always on the cutting edge, she pushed our faces into pornographic magazines and anatomy books to make sure that the human body would have no "mystique" for us.

The steady stream of negative comments about my father did decrease my respect for him. As he lost credibility with me, his ideas and concerns began to seem unimportant and any attempts at discipline ridiculous. We absorbed Ingeborg's negativity until we, too, resented him.

How he ever managed to raise us alone still mystifies me.

CHAPTER 5

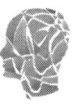

Just Desserts

"Ha!" I laughed as the belt came down on my rear. My dad had caught me reading Stephen King's *Carrie* with the light turned off in my bedroom. I was eight, just after getting expelled. "Ha-ha! It'll never work, Dad!" I taunted. It stung, but I knew his heart wasn't in it and that laughter was the best reaction to undermine his will. He was furious not because I was up reading, or because of what I was reading, but rather because I was reading without a good light and was wrecking my eyes.

Soon after, he moved me into my mother's old bedroom and gave me a reading light.

My new school was happy to have a bright young kid. Our teacher once asked the mayor to speak to our class, inviting the local press. "Fourth Graders Grill Maloney" ran the front page headline the next day, beside my photograph.

On the playground, though, some of the kids were not so happy with Mr. Smarty Pants. I had never learned how to defend myself, so when they came after me, I just kept backing up. Eventually I reached the chain-link fence, and one of them suddenly shoved me, hard.

"Think you're so smart, don't you?" he said. I instinctively reached to brace myself, sinking one of the sharp link tips into my right middle finger as it tightened around the pole. I felt pain and looked behind me: I was impaled on the wire.

"Hey!" I spun around, but the kids were running away. "Serves you right!" one of them yelled. I turned back to try to ease my finger off the wire, only causing more blood and pain. I screamed my throat hoarse, terrified I would never get loose.

It took some twenty minutes for the ambulance to arrive. My father was first on the scene, though, with bolt cutters. The school had called him at the laboratory where he was an engineer. This would not be the last time he would have to come to my rescue.

CHAPTER 6

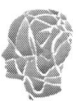

Dad Hosts the Mongol Horde

When my father was a boy, his family farm in East Germany had been occupied by the Soviets. One of the first actions of the incoming soldiers was to execute any remaining non-communists hiding from the revolution in Russia. My dad's parents had been sheltering a family from Ukraine; the soldiers killed them all, shooting each of them in the back of the head.

My dad and his brother had to bury the bodies of their neighbors.

The farm's quince trees were just starting to ripen at the time, filling the air with a tart smell. Every time the boys ached from the shoveling, the soldiers would push automatic weapons into their ribs and urge them on gruffly: "*Davai, davai!*" The Russian language, which my father had previously associated with the friendly couple living on the property, now came to mean horror and violence.

Mongols on ponies occupied his village, accompanied by a tank. The ponies were tied to a rail at the farm. The Mongols commandeered the main building. In the middle of the night, my dad and his older brother sneaked from their hiding place in the woods to see what the forces were doing in their home.

"There's a circle of their stuff in the dining room," said my dad's brother, peering in through the window. "No, it's them! They've flipped the chairs over and moved them into a circle. They're sleeping over the chair backs!"

There they were, face down and backs in the air, warm and dry on their makeshift chair-ponies in the dining room of my father's farmhouse. My dad and his brother sneaked back to the woods. First executions, then Mongols appropriating chair backs as mattresses. What could be next?

I found out about the executions only as an adult. The way Dad told it when I was a child, the gravedigging never figured in the story. According to the sanitized version told to regale guests, he and his brother decided to leave their homeland in high school when they were forced to learn Russian. "I found out we were the class enemy by reading Marx," he always used to say.

It made for an exciting tale. He escaped with his brother on the subway through Berlin before the wall was built, wearing two sets of clothes, one on top of the other, so at least he would have a clean set upon arrival. At the consulate he was encouraged to apply to American universities so he could emigrate and become a taxpayer. He chose MIT at random, was accepted, and was soon on his way, ignorant of the school's prestige.

When he came to the US, my father thought he had left concerns about Russia behind, but my curiosity would bring it up for him before long.

CHAPTER 7

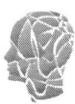

Saved by the Computer

"Can I go on the school trip to Moscow, Dad?" I stood at his bedroom door on the second floor of his house in 1979. I was in eighth grade. He was sitting in his leather swivel chair at his desk, hammering out correspondence on an electric typewriter.

"What do you plan to do there?" he asked, still typing.

"We're going to sell blue jeans on Red Square."

He slowly swiveled to look at me directly. "Why do you want to go?"

"Everyone else is going. The teacher says it will be educational for us to see another country." I was an academic star by now but socially felt pretty left out at school. I was no longer bullied, but I didn't have many friends, either. Maybe traveling together would let me bond with my class.

"Thomas, you're not safe there. You can't even read the signs!"

"Oh, c'mon, Dad, what about body language?"

"Thomas, you don't understand. Once when I was young, a drunk soldier almost shot me for not inflating his bicycle tire. You can't protect yourself if you don't know Russian."

Of course he was telling me a white lie. The bicycle tire was a metaphor for the gravedigging and the threatening Mongols. All I understood was that my popularity in class was going to stay low for another year.

"Please?"

"I'm not going to pay for any trip to Russia until you learn the language," he said. It seemed that I was the only kid in the class whose parents would not let him go.

I next turned to my mother for help with my loneliness. "Why does Julia get to go to private school and I have to stay in public, Mom?" I asked her once when we were alone in her apartment. "It's not fair."

Ingeborg looked at me for a long time. "No, you're right. It's not fair. Some things in life just are not fair." I knew that she was paying tuition and could make the decision to keep us together in public school.

"But Mom," I whined, "why?"

Rather than go into details, she relented, taking my sister out of private school as well, saving herself thousands of dollars, which she later donated to a human rights organization.

Since I had skipped a grade when I was expelled, Julia and I were in the same class. Two smart kids in the same grade made for fierce sibling rivalry. My sister, reporting now from the outside, wrote what I considered an arrogant column for the private school's newspaper during her first semester, titled "Teen Pregnancy and Drug Use in Wilmington Public Schools." In response, I championed the public school indignantly, writing a fuming column for our school's own newspaper: "Can't Read the Writing on the Wall?"

Sports were no part of my social life either, since doctors would not allow anything but swimming for me, a growing boy with a crooked back. But I did not make the swim team's cut. I spent most of my afternoons in high school hanging out, either online or in person, at the University of Delaware's computer lab. My room, otherwise a dump, was equipped with a Heathkit computer terminal my father had helped me build from scratch. For him, being a computer dad was less labor intensive than being a soccer mom, though it did mean I tied up the phone all afternoon and evening.

I envied a nerdy classmate who made regular weekly trips with the lab's coordinator to back up the system. His parents hadn't painfully split up. Maybe they had even given him the idea to do something constructive at the lab.

I, on the other hand, soon turned to delinquency. Some elder programmers, real adults, had been allowed online, and one of them, it became known, had written a short routine to crash the system. I had to give it a try. By that time, though, the administrators knew about the bug too and had implemented a booby trap. I was quickly found out.

Amazingly, I was forgiven without repercussions. My transgression was regarded as a learning experience.

***

"So, Tom, where do you see yourself in five years?" asked the admissions officer at the small Quaker college.

"I don't know," I said forthrightly.

"Well, what do you do for fun?"

I thought for a moment. "I was captain of my school's chess team," I said. "And I bicycled all the way around the Delaware Bay with my buddy once in high school." Somehow I never mentioned that I had instigated the crash of the university's computer network. More than biking or chess, I loved to program computers.

The college, Haverford, had an idyllic orientation period where freshmen got to know each other before academics began. One of my roommates wanted to become a rabbi, another a professor. Everyone but me seemed to have goals. At the end of orientation week, the admissions officer gave a talk to the incoming class. "If any of you are still not sure why you are here, come see me in my office," he concluded. Suddenly my heart warmed: I would be given a sense of purpose.

I knocked gingerly at his large wooden door. "So, Tom, we remember each other, don't we? Your sister called me to plead your case when you didn't get admitted on early decision. Let's see," he said, pulling open a drawer and searching for my file.

"Yes, I recall that you didn't have much of a sense of direction, but we thought we would give you a chance," he said, smiling.

My hopes fell. No sense of direction? My identity as a juvenile delinquent, as a "bug in the system," might well have been sealed by his pronouncement. But fortunately, in the late nineteenth century, a farseeing president of the college had instituted an honor code, making students answerable to themselves for their behavior. In practice this code often brought out the best in the college's self-selected students—and it would in me, too.

"Thanks, Bill," I said quietly, getting used to the Quaker custom of calling adults by their first names. I meandered through the dark hall, unlocked my bike, and pedaled home under the noontime sun.

I decided to stay at Haverford over Thanksgiving break, bicycling with Mark, a basketball jock from Baltimore who lived across the hall. I came home for Christmas but decided to stay at school for spring break, too, asserting my independence from home. After all, the dorm came equipped with a kitchen.

To my surprise, a large package from my father arrived over Easter. Sitting cross-legged on the kitchen floor where I had been eating iceberg-and-vinegar salad from a cast iron frying pan, I eagerly opened it to find a cake in the shape of a bunny. Our traditional holiday treat! For the first time I fully appreciated the extent to which he had been my caring provider for ten years. How could Ingeborg have turned me against him? I almost burst into tears.

CHAPTER 8

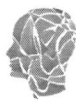

First Love

As I lay browsing the course catalogue the following term, I noticed a Russian class taught at Bryn Mawr, Haverford's sister school, where I was free to take classes. Five mornings a week for two semesters. It is astounding what children latch on to as challenges to overcome, usually from their parents. The chance to finally go to Russia on my dad's terms seemed within reach.

"*Ya. Ya nye. Nyet,*" I practiced aloud eagerly, listening to the cassette provided by my professor.

It was my sophomore year, and I had settled into school by rooming with Mark. "Could you keep down the harsh gutturals?" he joked.

"Mark, this language is so cool. One of their letters is *yo.*" The idea appealed to my adolescent mind.

The only requirement of the course was to practice every day. There was very little memorization involved, because my professor had been one of the first in the English-speaking world to systematize the language the way Latin is ordered. I thought I had hit the college jackpot with my background: Russian took the same kind of thinking as computers, meaning straight A's without any sweat.

It was 1985. College was starting to be fun. That year I even asked Mark what it would take for me to join the basketball team.

He turned serious. "Tom, it would take an incredible amount of a four-letter word. You don't like it very much."

"What's that, Mark?"

"Give it some thought, Tom. Starts with a 'w.'"

He knew me inside and out. Of course he meant "work," and he knew that, nice as I was, I was too lazy to subjugate myself to a coach if I could avoid it.

No longer wanting any part of basketball, I turned to volunteer work. I would be my own taskmaster. Outside the Cherry Street Quaker meetinghouse in Philadelphia stands a historical plaque: "Civilian Public Service: During W.W.II, some 12,000 men who were classified as conscientious objectors to war . . . served in non-military occupations across the United States . . ." I embraced my dignified new status and even volunteered for Philadelphia's Central Committee for Conscientious Objectors.

Gorbachev was not yet news. A Russian major would have meant a career in government or academics. I was not ready for the demands of either. Having successfully fumbled my way through college up to the middle of my sophomore year, I felt an impending sense of the "w" word.

"Dad, I think I'd like to take a year off," I told him at the kitchen table over spring break.

"Okay, Thomas, as long as you earn your own living. I don't want you to live here."

"Why not? I could fix meals for you. I make great salads."

"Thomas, you're on your own if you take a year off."

As usual, when my father laid down rules, I did my best to show him up. "Okay, Dad, if that's the way you want it." I sulked upstairs, lay down, and then was struck by a thought.

"Will you at least pay for summer school?" I poked my head into the kitchen again.

"In what?"

"Russian."

I can only imagine what went through his mind. "Okay," he said after a pause.

It's often said that most diseases have psychological roots. First my dad's German wife left him so he had to raise his children alone; then one of them was somehow attracted to the very country from which he had escaped as a child. That summer, my father had a heart attack.

At the time, I was helping to house-sit near campus. Only one of us, a country Quaker from North Carolina, was mature enough to make sure all the dishes got cleaned every evening. He dragged me out of bed for a phone call one night.

"What's up, Dad?" I asked, surprised to hear his voice.

"Thomas, I have to go to the hospital. If you need to, call the clerk of the Quaker meeting."

"Why would I need to do that, Dad?"

After a brief silence he mysteriously hung up. For a moment, a mild tremor shook the foundations of my world, maybe a two on the Richter scale—the thought of life without a safety net. A similar shock had hit when my mother left the house. But it passed more easily this time, caught up as I was in a routine of summer study.

My father survived the operation and stayed on to support me for many years longer. Somehow I couldn't get out of the routine of being a student, though. In the summer of 1988, after college, I studied German at the Goethe Institute in Düsseldorf.

I arrived complete with a bicycle and the fastest communications link to America I could afford: a portable typewriter. The Internet was not yet in common use and telephone calls were expensive. I was hatching plans with my college roommate for a bike trip through Russia and wanted to stay in touch.

I met Angela while peering over my handlebars, looking at a student bulletin board for accommodations cheaper than a hotel room. I still don't understand the appeal of young men on bicycles. "I could put you up until you find a place," she said, feigning disinterest.

As it turned out, I found my own place in university housing, but I eagerly took down her number. From then on, our courtship was innocent and sweet. After one hard day of study, I came home to a note on my typewriter: "As a matter of fact, Tom is rather a dumb cow." In German, this sounded cute.

Angela, a graduate student in biology at the university, was no farm animal herself. Later in the summer we bicycled together to visit Ingeborg's friend from high school. Neither my mom nor her friend had mentioned their hopes that I would fall in love with the friend's daughter, so as Angela and I made brilliant conversation over a cup of tea, I had no sense of foiling my mother's plans.

When we arrived back at the university dorm, we were tired and hungry. I remember turning to see her buxom figure backlit in the doorway of the kitchen where I was preparing us a quick meal. I felt an overwhelming desire to hold her. "Would you like to come to my place sometime?" she whispered in German.

I remember being so completely head over heels that when I returned to America, I called up my college girlfriend and asked her to meet me on campus. We sat on the grass together cross-legged, facing each other. "I met someone in Germany," I told her. "I'm in love."

Then I had my wisdom teeth pulled and was abandoned by my mother.

Had I had any sense, I would have flown straight back to Düsseldorf.

CHAPTER 9

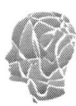

Heady Perestroika

In 1988, Russian studies had become quite the hot topic in America, what with Gorbachev and his efforts to reform communism. It seemed practical even for a pacifist to be studying the country. Since my timid freshman year, I had become goal oriented and driven, maybe even a little edgy.

To me, Russian studies meant visiting Russia in person, so I did, on a scholarship from an organization directed by my first-year professor. Pacifism? That meant actually doing something for peace, so I set about organizing an international exchange. Computers? I would figure out how they could teach Russian. Surprisingly, I had my father's support. My attraction for the country had turned him from a Russophobe into a Russophile.

I arrived in Moscow to study at the Pushkin Institute when I was twenty-one, bearing the name of a contact, Leonid. My father had hosted him in Wilmington one night when he visited as part of a delegation of peace walkers. I rang him up from the subway. Before leaving America I had been briefed in Moscow street smarts. Since private telephones could be so easily bugged by the KGB, the safest way to make calls was from busy public places.

Leonid was a privileged Muscovite. His office was in the main tower of Moscow University. When I inquired about the six unused beds pushed up against the walls of the spacious but poorly lit room, Leonid explained that his office had once been a communal apartment. A samovar on a nightstand made hot water for our tea.

"So, you want to arrange a bicycle exchange?" he asked, stroking his beard. "I think my son-in-law Misha can help. He has just become the new chairman of the Soviet Peace Committee."

To visit Misha, I needed to make a connection between a long subway ride and a bus. He met me with a broad grin at his door. "Take off your shoes, stay a while. Do you play chess?"

We were well matched. "So, Tom, which one of us shall go first on this peace exchange of ours?" Misha asked, advancing his bishop. His wife brought out a heavily creamed pasta dish for us.

"Your team, of course," I said guilelessly. I did not want to seem to have an agenda, and not asking to go first was the best way to demonstrate that I had none.

"Really?" he smiled. "Would you be willing to say that in front of the Soviet Peace Committee?"

"I don't know why not," I said confidently, advancing my queen a rank. "Check."

He interposed a piece. "Would you be willing to speak on Moscow radio, too?"

"Ha-ha, Misha. Do you think Muscovites are willing to listen to my bad Russian on their radios? If that's what it takes for me to be the first American to bicycle through their country, so be it." I took his piece.

"Wonderful," he said. "I never thought negotiating with an American would be so easy." I won the game.

I wasted no time incorporating my as-yet-unrealized peace initiative into my résumé, submitting it to the Pennsylvania Rhodes Scholarship Committee. Before long an invitation to interview arrived, forwarded from my Wilmington address, and I casually folded into my plans a quick return to the US for the interview, convinced against all odds that the scholarship was in my pocket.

During the same semester, still studying Russian at the Pushkin Institute, I pressed my teachers about computers and Russian. Eventually they relented. "There is a philologist at Moscow University who can answer any question you have about language," one of them said. "His name is Sergei Ivanovich Kiselev. He has written a small book that is very well regarded in some circles."

I was too lazy to invest long hours in reading the book before meeting its author, though. Used to relying on fast talk, I decided to crash his departmental committee meeting. When I intruded in sneakers and jeans, a woman was defending her thesis. I snuck to a corner and seated myself.

"And who is the American who has joined us?" the chairman asked playfully.

I started in boldly. "My name is Tom Hartmann, and I have a question about—"

"I will see you at home later tonight," he told me with a wave. He turned back to the candidate. "Please proceed." I was tapping into the certain cachet that Americans seemed to have in Gorbachev's Russia.

By semester's end, I had secured an agreement with a Soviet official, enjoyed office hours at home with a member of the intelligentsia, and been interviewed by the press. In a foreign country, I had actually managed to feel important.

Making an impression back home turned out to be a little harder.

CHAPTER 10

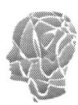

To Russia With Love

The Rhodes scholarship interviews were held at the University of Pennsylvania. I had arrived jet-lagged and sure of myself the previous night.

"So, Tom, tell us about your bike trip," one of my interviewers started off hopefully. The panel was grilling me in a small classroom at Penn's Wharton School for business. The scale of my ambitions to carry out citizen diplomacy had evidently piqued their interest.

I had vigorously promoted the exchange on my résumé, but it was really only in its planning stages. While typing my CV on the US-provided electric typewriters I found in Moscow, I had crammed it full of volunteer and extracurricular activities, hoping somehow to impress on them that I was in fact worthy of study at Oxford.

I wished I could have claimed to be an athlete, since I suspected that it would make me seem well rounded. Unfortunately, my scoliosis had kept me in a brace until just before high school, and even after that I only cycled and hiked—hardly participation in a team sport.

"Sure," I gulped, and said with bravado, "Just let me get some papers from my portfolio . . ." Fast talk and big words had always served me well in the past, but jetlag and mental haziness left me at a loss for words. Since when does a ratty backpack qualify as a portfolio? I was still thinking in Russian, using their term for briefcase: *portfel*.

I retired into a miserable silence to collect myself. When I tried to speak again, I saw in their eyes, kind and considerate as they were, that it was all over for me. Later, all six Pennsylvania semifinalists were called back into the office, and two were asked to stay. The rest of us were told, "Congratulations. We'll be watching your careers."

That was it! Dejected, I stepped out onto Locust Walk, feeling as if I had missed my chance to change the world and was that much closer to confronting hard work without any of the privileges that had paved my way so far.

I received another blow when, just after my interview in December, I learned that my roommate and the rest of the American team I had organized had lost interest in the bike trip and were backing out of their plans to join me. I needed to scramble to find a substitute leader and recruit willing participants. I found myself on the phone with the main US-Soviet exchange organization in Washington, DC, talking with Carter Fields, who turned out to be a fellow Haverford graduate.

"You don't happen to be a Quaker, do you?" I asked. This bond would only serve to strengthen my confidence in him.

"Well, as a matter of fact, I'm a member of Adelphi Friends Meeting in Maryland," he said. "I'm also an enthusiastic cyclist."

It sounded too good to be true, but the impending trip was near collapse and I was ready to do anything to save it. I had already seen that I couldn't count on student volunteers to be responsible, so I decided to hire Carter to coordinate plans while I finished up my second semester in Moscow. On the strength of his word, I sold my car to pay him before I left and hoped for the best.

That spring I fell in love with Tatiana, Sergei's stepdaughter. Angela, my German love, seemed so far away. Inclined to feel abandoned anyway, I was not sure she still cared for me.

Tatiana had a background very similar to my own: we were both directionless children of the Cold War generation who had been encouraged into academics for safekeeping from life's hardships. I met her when she was just finishing her graduate degree in Greek philology—not so odd a topic for an Eastern Orthodox country like Russia. Besides, her stepfather had helped write her thesis. Sergei had wooed Tatiana's beautiful mother away from her real father with his brilliance and persistence, even though he was some twenty years her senior.

"I would rather have studied business," Tatiana confided to me on one of our many evening walks near the river.

Once she came to my dorm and took care of me Russian style when I was sick, bringing wool socks and medicinal mustard plasters. A visit by a native Russian to foreigners from the West could only have happened in the changing political climate. The Iron Curtain was slowly opening. It was exciting, and she was beautiful. My suitemates pressed me for news about her after she was gone.

I knew that I somehow wanted to tie my life to hers—if not at Oxford, then somewhere else. When acceptance letters arrived that spring, I was admitted to two schools, the University of Wisconsin in Madison and New York City's Columbia. My decision was made for me: how would Tatiana, the big-city girl, ever be happy in Wisconsin, so far from a metropolis?

I decided on Columbia and invited my petite Russian girlfriend to come with me. Under the new regulations, travel abroad was now possible for Soviets with invitations. I was sure that study would come as easily as it always had. So my focus was elsewhere: maybe Tatiana and I would get married . . .

CHAPTER 11

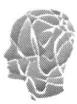

Cycling for Peace With the KGB

At the end of my spring semester in Moscow, instead of heading home with the rest of the American students, I delayed my flight until late August.

All that spring I had been planning the Russian leg of the bicycle exchange with Viktor, a professional outdoorsman Misha had found for me in Moscow. He was the Russian counterpart of Carter, the Quaker cyclist I had hired, except Viktor's reward for planning the trip was not the value of my car but rather the chance to see America for the first time.

A week later, I saw off the excited Russians from Viktor's apartment, feeling less certain than they did about how things would go during the upcoming month in America.

I spent the summer at Sergei's *dacha*, a country house near a muddy swimming hole a half hour's train ride from Moscow. He had designed the construction himself and had added a traditional Russian steambath toward the back of the property. He had even paid some townspeople to dig a private well outside the kitchen door. Everyone else used communal water.

At the time, life under Gorbachev was becoming chaotic. Reforms had brought about irreversible changes, and they were happening too quickly for any institution or person to digest them. Even the Pushkin Institute awarded me my diploma before I completed the coursework. I didn't complain.

When I returned to Moscow from the *dacha*, though, I discovered that Carter had facilitated something extraordinary through his connections in American Quakerdom: the team of cyclists had been hosted from Greenwich, Connecticut, to Washington, DC, by Friends meetings. The Russians were fed home cooking and put up in well-to-do houses, where Americans could not wait to meet them. I heard that Misha of the Soviet Peace Committee had celebrated his arrival in Washington by jumping from his bicycle into a public fountain, shouting, "I'm free!" and embarrassing his modest fellow countrymen with his flamboyance.

When Viktor and the other Russians returned from America, they brought with them three students and a hippie from Colorado, all wearing T-shirts emblazoned with "Cyclists for Peace" on the front in red, white, and blue. My brainchild, rejected so recently by the Rhodes panel, had become something exciting. I gained renewed confidence in my ability to turn ideas into realities.

Then-President Reagan's slogan "Trust, but verify" obviously applied to both America's and Russia's ways of handling the changes. When the second leg of the trip started in Northern Russia, we were "verified," too. "Hey," remarked one of the cyclists riding alongside me, "hasn't that big black car been following us for two hours now?"

Viktor smiled at him. "KGB agents. Don't worry. We have a pass from the vice-chairman. Anyway, they're just checking to make sure you really are American college students. Let me tell you, in those clothes, you sure do look the part." Our Yale graduate sported a brightly colored, skin-tight Lycra cycling outfit—something unheard of in Russia at the time—while I wore a white T-shirt and a helmet, a precaution that wouldn't have occurred to our counterparts. The car stopped following us around noon.

Our trip began north of Moscow and aimed west toward Leningrad, where we would turn south and pedal through the Baltic states before taking a train through Ukraine to the Crimea. From there we would travel again on our bicycles through the beautiful peninsula before boarding a boat that would take us across the Black Sea. The last leg of the trip would be through Georgia.

Throughout the trip, our group spent nights wherever we chose to stop—something new under Gorbachev. But you'd be naïve to think that the Soviets took chances: a KGB agent had been planted in our group.

He was athletic and friendly enough not to stand out, though. In fact, I never suspected him—it was our Yale graduate, skeptical about the Russians from the beginning, who first figured it out. Halfway through the trip he expressed a certain amount of distaste. After all, I had promised a no-holds-barred exchange.

After a day of cycling in Northern Russia, we paused at a ramshackle house with a beautiful flowering arbor near the road. I had often looked for flowers when judging potential rest stops in Pennsylvania's Lancaster County on biking trips during my college years. A World War II widow answered our knock and took in the sight of us.

"Sure, you're welcome to spend the night. I'm sorry, all I can offer you is the dining room floor," she told us. "But tell me, what brings you all the way out here? Isn't it nicer in America?"

"We came to see how real Russians live," I said. "They never taught us that in school." In fact, the Russians accompanying us were mostly engineers from Moscow and were almost as curious as I was.

That far north, keeping warm is vitally important. Like most peasants there, the woman had rigged up a bed on top of the centrally located stove, which would still be warm in the winter from the day's cooking. She kept her cow alive year round by housing it in the basement. We slept like sardines on her floor, only occasionally awakened by the rustlings of the animal.

We found our way to Leningrad with the help of Viktor and our handy KGB-provided maps. Ordinary civilian maps at the time were deliberately distorted in order to throw an enemy off course. Russia painfully remembered repeated invasions from European neighbors.

In Leningrad, talks had been arranged for us at an Orthodox seminary: religious tolerance was new under Gorbachev, and we were getting a full blast of openness. I enthusiastically talked about my own religion, Quakerism, and about pacifism. I was so idealistic at the time! The war-weary priests tolerantly listened to my youthful sentiments while the Yale graduate looked on skeptically. I knew the only reason he was with us rather than in the Air Force was bad vision.

Tatiana visited when we were staying near the Baltic Sea.

CHAPTER 12

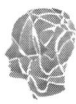

Bottoms Up

"Hey Tom, you guys want to be alone? I can go sleep in the bathroom tonight," my tentmate politely offered, anticipating the need for privacy often encountered among communists.

Tatiana, however, had already arranged a room with a local friend. She seemed to have connections everywhere, something that came from family background and schooling. In Russia, people cultivated their contacts more than they did in America: it had been a survival skill under communism.

Her family's prestige was cultural rather than political. Sergei had studied in the same graduate seminar as the chairman of the KGB. He was proud to be a communist, not for any selfish reasons but because workers had sheltered his father, a twelfth-generation Orthodox priest, from the revolution. He considered himself a conservative whose mission as a professor was to preserve a love of language and culture in the left-leaning Soviet state.

The Baltic Sea was too polluted for swimming, but it made for a romantic beach. Raising herself on her elbow to look at me, Tatiana said, "You know, you are getting quite the runaround here, compared to how the Russians were treated in America. The Quakers who met the Russians opened their hearts to them, and here you are being hosted by officials spouting the party line!" She was referring to some lightweight propaganda meetings Misha had been obliged to schedule for us.

From her vantage point in the Soviet Union's ivory tower, the events of perestroika that had motivated the exchange seemed like so much foam on the Baltic. "You're going to study political science? What's scientific about politics?" She fell back on the sand. Because of her family's connections, she had received a great education. And like her stepfather at the kitchen table, she felt sophisticated enough to toss off judgments about fields of study with which she was barely familiar. But I let it go. I was in love.

I didn't know what political science involved before entering graduate school; the field was just an adjunct to my Russian studies. As I talked with Tatiana, though, it seemed to me that I had sailed through Haverford's coursework without really understanding the country itself.

* * *

In the Crimea, our group was treated to breathtaking views of the Black Sea from cliff-hugging roads that switched back and forth to the shore. An American cyclist even dared to ride one of these stretches "no hands" in order to snap a picture of the vista from his bike. He grabbed his brakes just in time to avoid a crash with the next turn's rockface.

In Yalta, we boarded a cruise ship from the Crimea to Batumi in southern Georgia and enjoyed the good life, Soviet style.

The locals greeted us with figs and dates, the ancient equivalent of ice cream. We passed through rough-hewn mountain peaks, our progress impeded only by shepherds driving their flocks across the road. Georgian villages, even dirt-poor ones, met us with banquets every night. Once a piglet that ran between our spokes as we pulled in stared up at us from a dinner platter later on.

At first, this sort of hospitality was fun and welcome, and we indulged ourselves generously. But eventually the novelty began to wear off.

As we came over a crest in the Abkhazia region, the sight of soldiers with submachine guns made me feel queasy. I had not encountered real violence since the school playground. Viktor, cycling in the back, quickly sized up the situation and deployed our only defense tactic: a wide grin and a wave.

"These are cyclists from America!" he called. This was 1989, before Georgia became a pawn in a new Russian-American rivalry, and our country still had that special cachet. The men with guns were only local partisans in ragtag clothes and folded newspaper hats, checking cars for smuggled weapons. Tensions lifted as we posed with the guerrillas for photos. Innocence and goodwill proved a winning combination, something unusual in US-Soviet relations during the Cold War, but exactly what we had come to expect.

Our hangovers from the festivities eventually slowed us down. Early one morning after a particularly heavy night of eating and drinking, I and then another American ran to the outhouse to throw up the feast from the previous night and returned to sleep off our hangovers. Cycling thirty miles a day is one thing; covering that much mountainous terrain after repeated evenings of wild festivity is close to impossible.

Viktor came through for us once again. The Soviet Union at the time was still barely held together by its center, and we had KGB connections. Phone calls were placed to Moscow and arrangements quickly made at a local hospital for us to recover.

The chief doctor came to visit the ward where we lay. "Too much hospitality?" he asked with a smile. "Our people can be enthusiastic. We're so honored to have you here. Many of them haven't ever seen Americans in person before, you know." The Yale cyclist rolled to his side, away from the doctor.

"I wonder if you wouldn't let me apologize for our small nation, maybe with a little tea and chicken soup at my place?" We were not enthused. "Then we'll be expecting you!" My companion groaned.

Refusing hospitality in Georgia is a major affront. Not only were we the first Americans to visit this remote village, but we were also the first students on bicycles. Once we made it to the doctor's house we were greeted by yet another feast. It seemed that the entire town had turned out to meet us.

CHAPTER 13

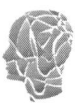

Marriage Without Mom

Even though we were still recovering from nonstop overindulgence, we did not have the heart to refuse eating again. Georgia's hospitality, as enjoyable as it invariably was, began to subtly impair our energy and focus. Viktor decided to call an early end to our exchange before real problems arose. Since Georgia was the final leg of the trip, calling it quits early didn't seem like a huge loss.

We had already seen almost every part of the western Soviet Union. Everyone we had encountered had warmly opened their homes to us, just like in rural Pennsylvania. Cyclists for Peace had abundantly fulfilled its mission of citizen diplomacy, for the summer of 1989 at least, and looked to a further exchange in 1990.

At the end of the summer, I asked Tatiana if she would join me in New York. For her it was a major life decision. Without really saying so, I implied that we would get married so she could stay for good. For someone like her, who knew little of the realities of a low-budget life in Manhattan, the offer must have been hard to refuse. She intended, with youthful determination and optimism, to somehow continue her studies of Byzantium in America.

Though we had only the money of my fellowship and the joyous approval of our parents—even of my father—I had no reason to think that my luck would end. My life seemed to have unfolded for me magically so far. On our small fixed income, we jumped into our life in the City together.

"They play chess just outside, on the sidewalk," explained Hope over dinner. Hope was an acquaintance in Columbia's administration that Tatiana had found through her enormous network of family contacts. I was pleased to have something I liked to do besides study, and Tatiana was delighted to arrive in New York well connected.

We lived in student housing on 112th Street near the Cathedral of Saint John the Divine. My approach had worked before: when I didn't know what to do next, I studied. The only difference now was that I was on track to becoming a high-powered professor.

Tatiana had a similar mindset. After all, she too came from a background that encouraged study, not work.

"Tom, do you think I'll get into Dumbarton Oaks?" We had recently toured that center for Byzantine studies in Washington, DC, while visiting one of the cyclists. She thought her prospects were good.

"I don't know, Tatiana. If it's like Russia, it's all about who you know, not what you know." Neither she nor her father knew anyone there.

Late in the fall, I wrote Sergei a letter in cursive Cyrillic asking for his stepdaughter's hand in marriage. Not only was I in love with the beautiful Russian at my side, but she also seemed the perfect match for me. Sergei was the intellectual giant that my parents had always wanted me to become and Tatiana's mother seemed to be the kind of loving, devoted homemaker I had been missing since age six. Finally, Tatiana was a charming conversationalist and companion who, at the same time, acted as a window into a culture that touched me deeply.

Sergei was delighted by my proposal. Like many Russians, he had an innate respect for my German background. He began to plan a career for me so I could follow in his academic footsteps. Tatiana's mother dealt with her departure by determining to visit us once a year in America.

At the time, I still saw Russia mostly through rose-tinted lenses, since my study under open-minded professors and my experience on the bike trip had reinforced my belief in the power of goodwill.

Tatiana and I were married in Wilmington in December of 1989. My father organized a reception in his own home. Even though he draped German, Soviet, and American flags on his side porch to make everyone feel welcome, the party lacked some essentials: Sergei and his wife couldn't afford tickets to come. What's worse, Ingeborg, still smarting from her divorce fifteen years before, boycotted the wedding.

A member of our Quaker meeting volunteered his house on the Jersey shore for our honeymoon, and one of our New York friends gave us a lottery ticket as a wedding present.

PART II

INTO THE ABYSS

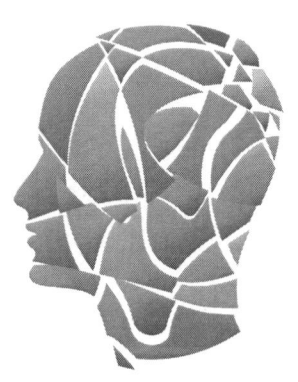

CHAPTER 14

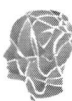

The Real World

"Tom, Hope says they're having the Blessing of the Animals tomorrow at the cathedral. Let's go, lovebird." Hope and her husband were one of our precious few links to life outside graduate school.

"I'm sorry, Tatiana, you go. Enjoy it for me." I was too preoccupied to really listen. The next day as I tramped by the cathedral on my way to the library, I passed the crowds with their dogs and cats, snakes and gerbils. I was wondering if I would find a good source for my next paper and was annoyed at the commotion. I had forgotten the excitement in Tatiana's eyes as she described the event.

I came home to find Tatiana reading a book. "Tomsik, let's watch Fellini tonight." She was no homemaker, but she knew how to spot a good movie. Both of us perused the critics' guides to videos carefully and watched anything that was well rated, snuggling together on a couch that Hope had found for us through a professor. Tatiana taught me to love films with subtitles. She had grown up seeing them through connections at Moscow's institute for cinematography.

We lived on a tiny budget, improvising meals from the local grocery in a wok every night and keeping leftovers for lunch the next day in a freezer my father had bought us when we first moved to New York. I ate a horse's breakfast every morning—raw oatmeal, walnuts, and cider—to keep me going until the afternoon. Ice cream was my one vice. Tatiana and I spread thin padding on the wooden floor and slept like Spartans.

We went to my father's house that year to celebrate Thanksgiving. An envelope addressed in familiar handwriting—Angela's—was waiting for me. "I will be on the East Coast soon, and could visit," my German girlfriend wrote. I put my tail between my legs. I had not meant to let her down by marrying Tatiana, but now I saw that I had made my choice. How to respond? I, who had left my college girlfriend for Angela, now had left her for a Russian wife. I could only be honest, I thought, and wrote her about Tatiana.

In the spring, Tatiana received a thin envelope from Dumbarton Oaks. She had not gotten in. When she got past her disappointment, Tatiana reluctantly decided to improve her already considerable command of English and pay for classes with earnings from a waitressing job.

"Tom, I don't like to work at that café," she announced after her first week. "I have to pretend to be grateful for such a small amount of money!"

"Oh, don't worry, it will only be for a little while. Soon I'll have a job and tenure, and both of us will be carefree," I said. In retrospect, I am amazed that this comforted her, if indeed it did.

The following semester we spent our free time together with our college friends, in Queens or across the Hudson in New Jersey. We often had dinner parties. Once a friend of Tatiana's, a Russian artist, captured the essence of the two of us in a line drawing. I subtitled it in Russian: "1988: Tatiana and Tom meet. 1989: The Berlin Wall comes down. 1990: The world breaks out in peace and happiness." I sent it around as a party invitation for her birthday.

The biggest disappointments we had encountered thus far had been not winning a prestigious scholarship, having to deal with temporary setbacks for the bike trip, and Tatiana's rejection from the top American school in her field. It never occurred to us that anything worse would be part of our otherwise promising lives.

CHAPTER 15

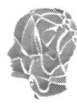

Deutschland

By spring semester, I was already in high gear. There is no such thing as summer break for a graduate student, just an opportunity for further study. I decided to apply for a scholarship in Germany, not to be closer to my relatives but simply for an excuse to study. Already edgy, I was losing perspective and becoming callous.

"I won't be gone long, Tatiana. Don't you think you'll have fun biking down the East Coast?" Cyclists for Peace, now in its second year, was the perfect opportunity for Tatiana to see America from the road. A new group of international cyclists pedaled from Burlington, Vermont, to rural Maryland while an American couple, one of them blind, rode a tandem bike through the USSR.

I joined the American contingent only in Philadelphia. One night we stayed on a farm near Pennsylvania's famous Lancaster County. "Why don't you two pose by the campfire?" asked one of the cyclists. I still have his photo: Tatiana's underlit face looks ghostly and distant. As soon as the exchange was over, I flew to Bavaria and Tatiana packed off to Wilmington to stay with my father.

By the summer of 1990, though, Gorbachev's novelty was already fading. The Russians were not so much impressed by America's hospitality as by its discount electronics stores. The moment for citizen diplomacy had passed, and that, more than anything, brought about the end of Cyclists for Peace.

When I applied for the scholarship in Bavaria, I had thought that I could brush up on my German and keep in touch with Tatiana by mail; everything would work out fine. I even thought that in my free time I would finish an overdue paper for which a professor had given me an extension. Surely, my darling wife would be happy in Wilmington.

"Sending you my tenderest feelings . . ." "I dream of us together . . ." Tatiana would write a postcard every single day I was away. On Mondays, more than one arrived. I wrote her a letter once a week. When I came back, I was so geared up that the next two semesters went by in a blur of research and long hours in the library.

In the spring of 1991, she addressed me with concern. "Tom . . ." I could hear trouble in her voice.

"What's going on, Tatiana?"

She looked into my eyes. "You know I am happy to be your wife, but put yourself in my shoes. This life in New York is not really what I had in mind when I came here. Being a waitress wouldn't be so bad if you were home sometimes, but instead you are always in the library or rushing around somewhere. Then you come home exhausted. Remember how it used to be? Two lovebirds? Free time in Moscow? It was so exciting at first, but that's not what's happening now, at least not for me. I'm really tired of it all. I want to get away. What if I were to spend the summer in Russia?"

"Yeah, I can see that would be great." As hard as I tried, I had no idea how to put myself in her shoes. "But you know," I added, "we could spend the summer in Wilmington. I haven't had much of a chance to see my father."

She gave a little snort. "I'm sick of Wilmington. It's so provincial and besides, your father charged me rent when I stayed with him all alone last summer. That's not the way to treat a family member!" That was true. It would never have happened in Russia.

"He can be like that, but—" I began.

"Tom, that's not the point!" she interrupted. I was surprised that she and I were so out of touch. Usually I could tune into what she was feeling just by watching her eyes. "My life is just so empty here!" She looked at me.

In fact I had not been giving her my full attention: part of my mind was on my next paper. I found myself standing there as if I were giving her problem some consideration, a pensive expression on my face, but with no ideas to go with it. I remembered the sound of her voice as she spoke, but the words didn't stay with me. My mind was racing, filled with images of the library, of my father, of college, of the cold weather, of the *dacha*, of her eyes scanning my face for some affirmation of whatever she had just said. "Exactly what do you mean?" I didn't want to say I had no idea and figured it would come to me if I just asked for clarification.

"Tom, life here means nothing to me anymore," she finally said, staring up at me firmly.

Suddenly I remembered the image on the birthday party invitation. The drawing showed me with a bicycle at my back, carrying Tatiana in my arms. She, in turn, was rubbing her eyes with her fists, as though she had been crying. Things began to come back into focus. "Waitressing, English classes . . .You really haven't been having a good time." She all but collapsed in my arms as I put them around her.

"You're right. Seeing your family would be a welcome change. For me, too." I wondered how I could have failed to notice that she had been so unhappy. Maybe she had not wanted to weigh me down with her problems while I was preparing for my oral exams the next fall. After all, half of the doctoral candidates failed them the first time. After a moment I added, "You know, I haven't taken a break since I began to study. A vacation will do me good, too. Let's just go. Together."

"Yes, Tom," she agreed. "You are a complete wreck. Let's go as soon as the term ends."

CHAPTER 16

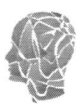

Over the Edge

Even though I had indeed been driving myself into the ground, I insisted on bringing study materials with me. Instead of the usual suitcases and gifts for the relatives, I dragged onto the plane a duffel bag of three cardboard file boxes full of academic journal articles. I was convinced that only if I mastered all of them could I hope to survive in graduate school. I wasn't able to conceive of a vacation without studying like a maniac.

Once we had arrived at Sergei's apartment, I dozed in a chair while Tatiana excitedly chatted with her mother and installed herself in the bedroom. I drifted off listening to their voices and soon fell into a profound sleep. Tatiana was shaking my arm when I awoke.

"Didn't you hear?" she asked. It was hard for me to wake up. "Come and eat. Mom has fixed your favorite—beet salad!"

I got up slowly and staggered to the table.

I had been looking forward to this moment for weeks. Now I was annoyed at how tired I was, almost too tired to have a conversation. I limited myself to answering questions and shoveling in the food. Tatiana gave me a quizzical look. Before long she suggested that I go to bed. She would stay up a little longer, but she walked me back to her room, where I undressed and flopped onto the mattress. She covered me tenderly.

"We can sleep late tomorrow morning," she assured me. "That nine-hour time difference is brutal. I'll join you in a few minutes."

For the next ten days I rested almost constantly, getting up only to pee or eat a bowl of oatmeal. Sergei and his wife began to think I was in a depression and started administering home remedies.

Russians treat most illnesses themselves without consulting a professional, since hospitals are overcrowded and often unsanitary: institutional bathrooms are usually holes in the floor, with raised footpads on either side. Doctors are called as a last resort when home remedies have failed. Sergei first tried administering a root dug up by musk deer during mating season, but it had no effect.

In retrospect, this should have served as a warning not to push any further, but since we all wanted results, and fast, he next tried ginseng, a stimulant he had gotten in vials from the Chinese embassy. Sergei, besides being a philologist, was one of the country's foremost China experts, and he profoundly respected Chinese culture. At least the embassy would be sure to have top-quality ginseng. A more appropriate step, perhaps, would have been to summon a Chinese doctor to accompany its administration with a diagnosis.

As it was, the new herb worked—like a sledgehammer on a vase. Now I was awake twenty-two hours a day and convinced that I knew the answers to all of the world's problems. An idealist by inclination, I wanted to start effecting change right away.

During my rides on public transportation, I would pull out the spiral notebook I kept in my jeans to scribble down ideas about how to achieve world peace. As the days went by, the notebook filled with quotes I had overheard from Sergei and increasingly simple diagrams of what needed to be done. Soon I was drawing overlapping circles and thinking my notes needed to be saved for my upcoming thesis.

I was ready with witty comebacks for guests—in Russian, no less—at the parties Tatiana and I attended. On one occasion, I knocked back a shot of strong alcohol, Russian style, and my mind, already flailing in a sea of herbal concoctions, drowned.

As I fell under the influence, I quieted down and started to notice what was around me. I gazed at the cut crystal dangling from the chandelier. Flames seemed to dance in each facet, up in midair, floating below the ceiling. The reflected light was magically alive somehow. Hanging on either side of a mirror were two portraits. I studied them, sensing their significance.

At my knees was the hostess's dog. What a fascinating animal! Our eyes met. I felt the dog and I were old intimates. Stonehenge? Would I accompany him secretly there to obtain some important information? He wanted me to come into the hall to discuss it. I made a discreet exit. While we were conferring, Tatiana came in from the dining room to check if I was all right. She was concerned that the alcohol might have made me sick.

"Tanya," I confided, "we have an important trip to arrange as soon as possible." I could see she was confused. I began to explain, but she didn't seem to understand. Instead she coaxed me back into the dining room and suggested that perhaps we should be going.

I, meanwhile, had lost track of the dog and my mission. Confused, I allowed myself to be corralled into a taxi. I fidgeted in the back seat until we reached the apartment.

In the car, I sensed that something awful was about to descend upon us, a feeling of dread that I didn't recognize. The sensation had no distinct beginning, so I didn't have a chance to agonize as I saw it coming. On the other hand, I wasn't able to assess it in retrospect because it had no distinct ending either. Whatever it was, its intensity was unnerving, almost disgusting. There was no getting away from it. On and on it came. I couldn't even really sleep.

CHAPTER 17

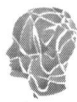

Fairy Tales

I dozed until just before dawn, waking up with the same awful sense of terrifying, hurtling reality. As the hangover wore off, I began to get used to feeling this way. Increasingly it seemed as if my state of consciousness was the enemy, and I wanted victory over it.

I ran into the corridor wearing nothing but a T-shirt, yelling at Tatiana. "I don't *want* to come back to bed!" Wide awake, I was obsessed with the fact, still new to me at the time, that I no longer had control over my thoughts and emotions.

It appears that I had been not only drunk, but also psychotic—and that I was still psychotic. A Western psychiatrist guessed many years later that I was experiencing my first full-blown manic attack, complicated by toxic psychosis. Insanity allows for moments of remarkable lucidity, and I was experiencing one just then: I remembered how it felt to be stable and desperately wanted that condition for myself again.

"No! No!" I yelled, in a voice no longer my own. I growled deeply, like something wild. To accentuate my refusal, I stamped my bare foot with bruising force against the thinly carpeted concrete floors of the Stalin-era apartment, but noticed no particular pain.

Soon my in-laws had called in a psychiatric emergency crew to sedate me and take me to a hospital. The men were actually wearing white coats. I wanted to hang on to whatever consciousness was left in me and, terrified of their needle, screamed as they approached.

Tatiana was torn apart by the scene; she knew that the medicine would do me good, but did not want to see it forced on me. She dismissed the crew before they gave me the shot.

Out of sympathy for my plight, Sergei, who knew me in my normal state, decided on a "philological approach." He, who could read over twenty European languages, gently invited me to rest a while under the covers where he slept. Even though I was lost in confusion, I responded and climbed into his bed as though mesmerized. On some level, I was probably recalling how I climbed into bed with my father after childhood nightmares.

Sergei was a great believer in the power of language, as the many books that virtually papered the walls of his apartment testified. He took down a book of Russian fairy tales and began to read in a playful voice.

Many of the words he read were unusual in everyday speech, but I could make out their general meaning. They ended in silly little sounds that rhymed with each other. In these tales the tsar referred to his subjects as children, and they, in return, called him "Grandpa."

I could not really follow the stories, but their overall effect did relax me. I had been too wired and overworked. For a moment, I took a rest, and eventually I fell asleep.

That day, unconscious on the bed, I spoke Russian without an accent, in a voice much deeper than my own. Tatiana said later that it resembled World War II soldier slang and her mother marveled that such a thing was possible. "Was Tom a channel for some departed soul?" they wondered.

After I awoke, time, once so seamless, began to have missing segments. I would, for example, continue a conversation from hours or days prior, as though I were answering a question that was hanging fresh in the air. It was as if my mind, stretched too taut, began to rip and tear into sections and could no longer cover the entirety of events. It applied itself to only parts of reality.

As a result, I began to speak increasing nonsense. I no longer remember exactly what happened after the fairy tale episode, although I am told that I continued to speak, respond, and move like a conscious person. My behavior was wild when I felt threatened with violence but otherwise responsive to gentle and persuasive words. Tatiana's mother and father finally took me to the hospital after home treatment proved hopeless.

Through Tatiana's high-placed friends, and only through those connections, I was admitted to Moscow's best psychiatric hospital for non–party members, an academic research facility.

CHAPTER 18

Shock Therapy

"I'm so concerned for Tom. What a nightmare!"

Tatiana and her family waited to speak to the night nurse in the admissions office. I had been packed off to a locked ward, sedated, and tied to a stretcher.

"At least they won't use violence at this hospital." All of them were aware of the brutal practices in most Russian mental wards, but in the almost surreal atmosphere of the makeshift waiting room, it was hard to take comfort from the thought that this institution wasn't quite as bad.

They all stood anxiously as the nurse in charge bustled into the room. She pulled out a clipboard and squinted. "The patient is an American. You are familiar with his case?"

"He has never displayed these symptoms on prior visits to Russia. He is my son-in-law. First, he slept almost constantly. Most recently, he seems to have an altered perception of reality. He has been in our country for about two weeks." There was relatively little paperwork and soon they were making an uneasy departure.

If the doctors had heard clues like "mood swings," "random thoughts," and "grandiosity," they might have diagnosed me as bipolar. In that case, they would have put me on the standard treatment, even in Russia, for manic depression—lithium. But, perhaps in an attempt to make sure things were under control, they guessed schizophrenia and prescribed a heavy-duty antipsychotic that left me with only a hazy window on life.

Every time the sedative began to wear off, I became enraged at my situation and the functioning of my mind. At this point, although the hallucinations had subsided, my thinking, surely the most powerful aspect of my self-image, was hopelessly clouded and my balance so poor that I was often reduced to crawling just to get to the bathroom or the dining area.

In response to my angry screams, the male nurse would be back to tie me to the bed. "Yes . . . ?" taunted one mustachioed aide as he routinely snapped bolt cutters dangerously close to my genitals once I was tied down. He would grimace as I stopped midscream and rolled my eyes, my jaw falling slack.

I grew scared and lonely. Always terrible at keeping myself company, I felt even more abandoned on the foreign hospital ward. The Russian psychiatrists made no effort to spend any time getting to know me; in fact, they seemed to cultivate an air of indifference. Visits from friends, including some of my Russian cycling companions, went a long way toward convincing me that I was still human.

"What's the news outside the hospital?" I asked Viktor's athletic wife once when she visited, bearing a homemade fruit salad.

"Oh, don't worry. Nothing really important: the government is being overthrown. Here, have some more fruit." In fact, Yeltsin's coup was imminent, but I, the political science major, had things more pressing to deal with, as she well knew.

Most of the time I was lucid enough to remember who I was: a native of Wilmington, Delaware, with Quaker roots. Would I ever get out of this hell and go home?

"Tatiana," I asked during one of her visits, "do you have a piece of paper, even a napkin that I could write on?" She could see I was agitated.

"Certainly, my dear." Institutional napkins were not very absorbent. Like Soviet toilet tissue, they had the feel of what in the West would be considered corrugated airmail paper. She found one and offered it to me with a pen. Scrawling a confused plea to my father, I asked her to convey it to him somehow.

My thoughts were too dim for me to envision what would become of my note. It was a message in a bottle: "Dear Dad, I am not quite sure what has happened to me, but I think it may have something to do with my childhood. I think the best place to sort these things out would be back at home. Love, Tom."

It didn't occur to me to contact my mother.

I awoke late the next day, still sedated. My awareness had dimmed for eight hours or so, but I had not actually ever gone to sleep.

Two patients who worked as staff assistants were sitting on a nearby cot. Shortly before, I had been aware of them leading a swarthy young Azerbaijani off the ward to the electroshock-therapy room. It was a privilege for patients to be entrusted with responsibilities, and like all Soviet-era hospitals, this one was always short on help.

"You don't remember, do you?" Dima, the broad-faced one, was asking.

Remember? No, I didn't remember.

"Last night, he punched you in the face. Too much medicine!"

So that was why the Azerbaijani had been seething and shaking his fist at me, I thought in an unfocused way. Yes, too much medicine.

Soon they fetched him, carrying his body by the shoulders and feet and dumping him like a sack of potatoes onto his bed. He would wake up in a few hours and, ideally, not remember a thing.

That day the doctors took me off bed rest and allowed me to roam the hall. As I wandered by, I noticed that patients had gathered to smoke in an alcove to the left, just across from the shock-therapy room. Dima and his buddy were sitting there. "Tom!" he called. Their fellowship enticed me, even though I did not know either one.

Smiling invitingly, Dima offered me a cigarette. I found out later that he played in a famous Soviet rock band. Not being familiar with Russian pop culture, I was not starstruck, and in any case, he did not flaunt his fame. Nonetheless, his presence on the ward spoke to the fact that the institute accepted only elite patients. I was there by virtue of my connections. Sergei had, after all, studied alongside the KGB chairman. Lucky.

Dima had manic depression. He was one of the few patients whose variant of the illness could not be treated with drugs. He lost his mind regularly. He knew his sickness well and had grown used to mental hospitals. He was familiar with this one in particular and the staff knew him.

I took his cigarette. I had never smoked but decided to make an exception for the occasion. I didn't even know how to take a drag. From watching other people, I knew how to hold it and how to accept a light, but I was mystified about what to do when I put it in my mouth. "How did you get here?" Dima asked.

"Well, I was on my father-in-law's bed, then I was jumping around the apartment, then everything just went black." I tried to look casual as I tapped the ashes off my cigarette.

The group murmured in agreement. "Went black—that's just how it is," said Dima. We sat thoughtfully. Then I began to extinguish the cigarette on the fleshy part of my knee.

CHAPTER 19

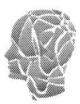

Nyet!

"What are you doing, lad?" Dima exclaimed. He grabbed my arm and wiped the ashes off my leg. A small red circle remained. I felt a sensation, but not very acutely. Dima led me out of the room and forcefully directed my limp body back onto the ward.

"Just lie here for a while; you'll feel better." He ran to get a nurse. I lay in the bed. Interesting events were happening. I was more stimulated than when I had been tied to the cot and was enjoying my freedom. Evidently the doctors needed to experiment more to get my medications right.

My case must have posed a challenge to them. I was experiencing my first episode—severe, and with no prior symptoms besides overwork. From the medical records I saw later, they never recognized that I had Chinese herbs and alcohol in my system. Small wonder they thought I was having a nervous breakdown.

In Russia, I missed out on what can be the tender side of psychiatry, maybe because of the huge language barrier. My doctors did not establish any rapport with me. They were not kind people, just strangers. In fact, when one of Tatiana's friends came to visit wearing a doctor's outfit as a joke, I screamed in horror.

Eventually I was allowed to visit the smoking alcove a second time. I had been switched to a different bed, in a private room, since I was still occasionally being assaulted on the general ward. Also, I began to run what was diagnosed as "brain fever"— meningitis, a rare drug side effect. The thin casing surrounding my brain was inflamed.

Again Dima hesitatingly offered me a cigarette. They probably did not invite me without some fear of the consequences. My nurse, bearing an eerie resemblance to the evil Nurse Ratched in the book *One Flew Over the Cuckoo's Nest*, had chewed them out last time, as though my injury had been their fault.

"Want a light?" Dima asked.

When he had pulled me to bed after my last visit to the alcove, he had been performing a nurse's duty and had been reprimanded. "Nurse Ratched" kept not only a strict appearance but also severe order on the floor. As I lit up, everyone watched me, the insane American, with a certain tense expectation.

This time, before taking a drag, I opened my mouth, stuck out my tongue, and extinguished the cigarette on the extended surface. The room cleared instantly, chairs crashing and patients tripping over each other to get out. I suppose they all wanted to be able to claim they were not present this time.

In fact, the cigarette left no trace, my tongue being moist. I only tasted ash, which I then tried my best to spit out on the floor. Despite the camaraderie symbolized by the cigarette, I guess that on some level I wanted to punish myself for accepting it. After all, I had never approved of smoking.

To address the meningitis, the doctors began a course of electroconvulsive therapy (ECT). This is not the standard cure in Western psychiatry, but in Russia, many things are different. I was strapped to a dolly and given regular jolts of electricity through my temples. To achieve a similar effect, the ancient Greeks used to surprise patients by unexpectedly pushing them from a near-deadly height into a pool of water.

Unfortunately, I reacted poorly to this cure, because in my mind ECT was associated with a lobotomy. After all, the hero of *Cuckoo's Nest* ends up with part of his brain removed. In effect brainwashed by the famous book, I thought that its plot reflected reality, having heard about it so often from my college roommate when he was writing a paper.

Patients are not supposed to remember their sessions of ECT. I do not remember my first and second convulsions, having learned about them only later from my medical records. But for better or worse I remember my third session: cold conducting grease being rubbed on my temples in an antiseptic room and a football-type guard being inserted into my mouth so that I would not bite my tongue or break my teeth when the current passed through my brain.

Inspired by one of the characters in the book, I decided to escape from the hospital and make it to Tatiana's by public transportation. It was too scary inside that place.

During a semi-wakeful moment in the middle of the night after the third session, I perceived myself as the king on a chessboard in a seriously compromised position. With the focused attention that I was still sometimes capable of, I scanned the room for any means of escape. My eyes finally fell on the top half of the two-panel window, not covered by bars. This was a mere academic research hospital, after all.

I vaulted myself over the top and hung from the outside of the window with no thought to the length of the drop. Nurse Ratched must have heard my scuffling and entered the room just in time to clap her hands to her cheeks and cry, "No, my son!"

I let go because I feared more for my life inside the hospital than out of it.

CHAPTER 20

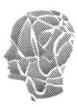

Desantnik

Fortunately, my room was only on the second floor. I broke my back, fracturing one vertebra in two places. I tried to crawl to the subway but could not move. A crew from the ward soon came to retrieve me.

My medical records do not show the further course of the meningitis. My guess is that they had pulled that diagnosis out of a hat. At any rate, the main concern became how to deal with my back. Their solution: tie me to the bed, this time permanently, back in the communal ward.

Tatiana, at her wits' end, finally called my father for help. When she phoned, he was on vacation in Big Sur. His house sitter was not able to get through to him at Esalen Institute, because that resort ensures the relaxation of its visitors by minimizing communication with the outside world.

Eventually, after receiving a desperate call from the house sitter, the local police pinned a handwritten message to a bulletin board by the hot tubs, where my father said he almost overlooked it.

The note was a masterpiece of understatement: "Hans Hartmann: Your son has broken his back in Moscow. Please come."

My father got on the next plane home. Familiar with the pressures of escape from communism as a young man, he was not willing to entrust my evacuation to embassy bureaucrats.

"Is this Carter?" Somewhere he had found the number of my Haverford cycling friend, who still worked at the US-Soviet agency in Washington. Together they arranged tickets to Moscow, and then my father worked out the details of the rescue as best he could. His greatest concern was how I would fit into a plane's tight coach seating in a full body cast.

He arrived in August of 1991, just days before Boris Yeltsin's coup. Awakened by the squeaking rumble of tanks as they made their way into the center of the city, he got up with misgivings and joined Tatiana's mother at the kitchen table.

"I had hoped I would never hear Soviet tanks again in my life. Sounds bring back memories, maybe more than any other sense. What grim days those were at the end of the war."

She kept her cool, saying, "The main thing is to get Tom home safely. The tanks are probably just for show." Soviets were used to military parades in their city streets. Sitting around the table, the family planned a rescue mission that involved obtaining plane tickets and getting me and my broken back out of the country.

Tatiana escorted my father into Moscow's city center to arrange exit papers. Genuinely frightened by the sight of a tank at the subway entrance, he turned to Tatiana for help and was surprised to see relief on her face. "Thank God," she said, "those boys are my classmates!" She talked her way past.

Later, faced with a crowd surrounding the US embassy, she thrust twenty-dollar bills into a taxi driver's hands and told him to keep pushing through the throng on the street. People crushed around the vehicle, glaring at us and knocking their index fingers against their temples in the European sign for "Are you crazy?"

The mental hospital wasn't equipped to handle major injuries. I remember riding on a stretcher across Moscow to another hospital's emergency room for an x-ray and cast.

The public vehicle that served as an ambulance was so poorly maintained that it was no more than a jalopy. Thanks to its poor suspension, I felt every bump in the road painfully, and the driver, in typical Russian fashion, thought nothing of running lights, whipping around corners, and sitting on his horn.

I was still dazed and moaned gratefully as my father squeezed my hand. "Don't worry, Thomas, this is the last step. Once your back is set, we can go home." His voice sounded especially sweet to me at that moment. Tied to the stretcher, I couldn't move to brush tears from my cheeks, but my father tenderly wiped them away.

"Breathe out." The nurse was wrapping warm plaster around my midsection up to my armpits, making an old-fashioned cast, the kind your friends sign their names on. Obediently I exhaled fully. Big mistake. Once the cast hardened it was so tight that I couldn't completely fill my lungs, but at least my back was secure. When the cast finally came off a week later, it seemed as if the muscles of my chest had shriveled. Free breathing took a while coming back.

We were more relaxed on the return trip to the mental hospital. My father described the sight of barbed wire—a remnant of Yeltsin's recent coup—to me as we passed the parliament building, and spoke of our imminent departure from Russia.

Back at the psychiatric facility, the arrival of my handsome and capable German father reduced Nurse Ratched's domineering style to petty groveling. On my last night, she woke me, urgently whispering, "You must take me with you! You need me!" I assumed she just wanted a ticket out of Russia and ignored her.

Later Dima came up to my cot and put his hand on my shoulder. "Eh, *desantnik*," he said, using the Russian word for paratrooper. "Looks like you made it out."

I put my hand on his and squeezed it.

Eventually my father, Tatiana, and I were accompanied by an uncle to the airport, where one of her cousins, a former Soviet marine, held a job at the customs desk. Connections, connections. With documents spilling from a billfold, the cousin took charge of a gate and ordered my father to find an American official to stamp some of the papers. Documents, documents.

My father seized the first uniformed American he could find and pursued him to another part of the airport, where he finally cornered him in an elevator. When the official ignored his pleas as a fellow countryman, he resorted to an appeal, father to father. "What would you do?" he asked. "My son needs Western medical attention and this is one of the last flights out of Moscow." He eventually got the official to accompany him.

"It appears that this man in the body cast will not fit into any of the seats in coach." One of the airline employees was conversing with his superior and pointing to me. "Is there still room left in first class?" Luckily we were close to the front of the line; first class sold out very shortly thereafter.

As always, everyone sat waiting in the plane for much longer than seemed necessary, but eventually we were settled and ready to taxi. Just as my father relaxed with a glass of champagne, my dependence on the medication kicked in and I went into withdrawal, vomiting all over my seat, fouling the first class compartment at the beginning of a ten-hour trip.

"Would any doctor on board please come to the first class compartment," announced a stewardess over the speaker system.

Within minutes at least eight men and women were streaming up the aisles and trying to push through the door from coach, each with a different opinion. Some peeked over the shoulders of those who had arrived first. They were all Soviet Jews taking what might be their last chance to leave the country.

The bearded captain descended the spiral staircase of the 747 to inquire into the commotion. "Do I need to turn this plane back around to Moscow?" he asked. My father took him aside for another man-to-man chat: "This is my son. I came all the way from America to save him."

An elderly female doctor had seen my sort of withdrawal before. After looking at my papers and medicines, she gave me the proper injection so that I would not have problems for the rest of the flight. "Everything under control?" the captain asked. When the doctor assented, he returned to the cockpit.

On our arrival at Kennedy Airport hours later, I felt sensitive to every stimulus: noise, light, touch, even thoughts and emotions. My hair stood on end from not having been washed for weeks. "Can you get up, Tom?" my father asked me gently as I sat in the plane, the last passenger to disembark. "No . . ." I murmured, more out of an aversion to any sort of contact than from a real inability to move.

Soon a steward brought a wheelchair and I allowed the staff to roll me into it, my full body plaster cast making the transfer particularly difficult. I moved like an enormous snapping turtle, long and solid in the middle.

By the time we deplaned, the stewardesses had long since finished bidding passengers farewell and had taken up different duties for the next flight. My father rolled me over the bump of the tunnel connecting the plane to the airport building. We were in America.

CHAPTER 21

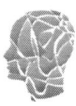

Homeward

The living chaos of the surrounding crowds assaulted my senses. Had I been faking insanity as my wheelchair rolled through JFK's lobby, I could hardly have done a better job. I lolled my head, held my hands over my ears, and moaned to my father to please slow down. I had not shaved since I jumped out of the window five days earlier. I wore dirty sweatpants, the same that I had lived in day and night at the hospital. In-flight eyeshades still covered my eyes.

My wild appearance caused even New York's busy airport crowd to give me a wide berth, like a stream around a protruding rock. We made our way quickly to the customs desk, usually the slowest routine of an international flight.

"He needs to get to a hospital soon," my father explained to the official. I moaned as if on cue, asking for him to slow down and begging for more medication. The customs officer cleared us quickly.

"Wait here. You'll be all right?" My father ran to get the car, leaving Tatiana and me on the pavement outside the arrivals terminal. The delay was excruciating. I felt like an angry dog being held in check—every moment was a tug on the leash. "Tatiana, I can feel those bugs under my cast again," I whined, "like on the plane. Maybe I'm going to throw up."

I alternately wanted to scream in desperation, pound the arm of my wheelchair, and tear at the plaster cast, which by now felt like a pressure cooker. I was going into withdrawal.

Restraining myself took energy and concentration. Babbling and insisting that no one touch or talk to me, I saw it as my family's job to get me home. In return, I thought, I would make no trouble. Actually, maybe just a little bit of trouble, only if necessary.

Tatiana waited with me at the busy curbside while my father got the car. She was forcing herself into a major life decision. She would stay in America and stand by me. Her stepfather had given her a stern lecture before her departure: "All people face difficulties in their lives. I faced mine during the siege of Leningrad, hiding from the bombing under the family piano and eating boot leather to survive. You'll survive too."

The New York City summer was in its final month and felt hotter and more humid than Moscow's. My body, gradually warming up after the air-conditioned lobby of the airport, became even more uncomfortable under the wads of cotton and plaster. I had been convinced that it couldn't get worse, but the sun seemed closer in New York than it had in Moscow. I felt my nose and cheeks getting hot, as though from a burn.

"Where's Dad?" I moaned to Tatiana as soon as he left. She took my hand and stroked it. "Don't worry, Tom. He'll be here soon."

By the time he swung in behind some taxis, I passionately wanted to get in the air-conditioned car. "Here, recline that passenger seat so he can roll onto it." They both helped me into the car, picking me up and shoving my cast in, then closing the door quickly.

"I'll get in back." It was Tatiana's usual fate, as a small woman, to tuck in behind the two tall men of her American family. The coolness in the car served to lower tensions a bit. My father had found New York's classical music station on the radio.

"Ahhhh! Dad, this car is a dream after the past couple of weeks." I closed my eyes and tried to exhale slowly. I still couldn't breathe deeply thanks to the body cast, but so many welcome sensations greeted me that I let complaints about my constricted breathing go and focused on my other perceptions instead.

"The feel of the velour . . . the angle of the seats . . . mmmm . . . the way it smells . . . the music . . . and it's so clean! It's just the way it always was. Maybe I'm not really insane!" Couldn't it have just been culture shock?

"We'll have to see," my father was saying. My thoughts snapped back from their musings about the car. No, it wasn't just culture shock. There they were: bugs crawling under my skin, pushing for a way out of the full body cast. And I still wanted the serenity the eyeshades gave me. The bright light hurt.

The drive to Wilmington from New York took several hours. By late afternoon, I was extremely agitated. I could no longer tolerate the close space of the car. Familiar with the route, I knew the distance home from the airport, but I let out my frustration in a stream of complaints:

"Dad, I think I need a new injection."

"Dad, when will we be there?"

"Dad, I'm going to get better, right?"

My father had no personal friends in the medical profession, but he had the mind of an engineer and knew how to handle a problem. "The most important thing is to be calm and take it one step at a time," he said, his eyes fixed on the road ahead. "If we can just keep our minds clear, we'll be able to see how to get from Point A to Point B."

Later, when I again expressed doubt, he told us, "Our biggest mistake would be to lose confidence. Answers are sure to come to us." He managed to reassure me; I don't know to what extent he reassured himself. I didn't hear him mention concerns about what he would do next to handle his career, his home, and his son in the coming days, and, no surprise, I wasn't worrying about any of those things either.

"Try to make it home, Tom."

"We'll be there soon."

"We'll get you better, Tom."

I tried to keep myself under control by remaining completely quiet and putting all my energy into fighting desires to scream and lash out. That job kept me from noticing time as it passed. Meanwhile, Tatiana gazed out the window of the car as if she were wondering exactly what sort of man she was married to now, and what awaited her in Wilmington.

"Careful on those steps, Thomas! You're not steady in that body cast," my father called. By the end of our trip, I had become unnaturally agitated. Excited to be home, I was heaving myself up and down the stairs inside the house, looking around at the changes my father had made.

He and Tatiana were preparing a favorite meal, chicken and mushroom stir-fry. So that's what he had run into the store for while I was agonizing in the supermarket lot. It smelled great, but I had no patience for a sit-down dinner.

"Where are you going, Tom?" my father asked.

"I want to visit the swimming hole down in Brandywine Park." I was still suffering from compulsive agitation as a side effect of my antipsychotic. Now that I had remembered the swimming hole, the thought of how I used to cool off with my childhood buddy gripped me and would not let go.

The round trip would take about forty minutes, even without the body cast. Although dinner was almost ready, I wasn't concerned, since in my condition I didn't feel hunger.

"Why don't you wait until you've had something to eat?" my father asked. Rather than making a fuss, I agreed. Being cooperative was an effort for me, but I was pleased to see my father's relief.

In childhood, I would have at least chopped vegetables for the salad, but now I made no effort to help out. I sat down at the kitchen table and waited to be served.

"How about helping set the table, Tom?"

"Oh. Okay." I scattered bunches of forks and knives by each plate and gave everyone a mug to save myself the effort of finding glassware. "There." Feeling jumpy, I suddenly dashed out of the kitchen, loped upstairs to my old bedroom, and curled up as best I could in a body cast, moaning and rocking back and forth.

"Thomas, are you all right? Let's all eat together, the way we always do. You haven't been home for so long . . ." I had been counting on him to come up and find me. It was true, eating separately in our household was just not done, but I couldn't come with him. I was in withdrawal by now, lying on the floor of my childhood bedroom, alternately lashing out with one hand and slapping the carpet, then clenching my fist and holding it against my forehead, moaning again. My leg was twitching.

CHAPTER 22

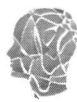

The Pear Cure

Perhaps Nurse Ratched should have joined me after all. My father knelt and put his hand on my shoulder, uncertain about the withdrawal reactions. "Come and have some food, Tom," he suggested gently.

I felt no hunger but didn't want to admit it. The unfamiliar body sensations I was experiencing made it hard to formulate a thought. "No—" I said, but didn't finish. A convulsion jerked through my body.

My father wanted me near him in case something else unexpected happened. "I'll help you downstairs. You can lie on the big carpet by the kitchen." I summoned the energy to get up and limped slowly down the steps, hunched as though wounded, as he followed me. I collapsed on the living room rug opposite the kitchen and watched through the door as he and Tatiana ate.

My dad worked a full-time job at DuPont but had decided to take time off until I stabilized. He was my twenty-four-hour watch, sleeping with me on the living room floor. Our first night, I awoke around 2 a.m., suddenly animated. I rolled free of my father's grasp and looked at his tired face. He was sixty-two years old and sound asleep.

"Dad," I whispered intently, looking at him.

He snored.

"Dad," I insisted, adding some voice to my breath.

He jerked awake, looking for a moment as if he were not sure where he lay. Then he focused his eyes on me. His eyelids were still drooping as he reached to pet my head. "How are you, Tomchen?"

"I'm hungry," I said, as though it were his problem. "I want a pear. A pear will cure me, Dad." The thought had seized me in the same manic way as had my visions of the swimming hole. I was focused on it now as if it held the key to life.

With very few exceptions, my father had given me his unconditional support. It was no different now, even though he knew that I was insane. Maybe he was working on the principle that "if treated as sane, he will begin to act sane." Or maybe he had a middle-of-the-night association with pears, the quince trees of his youth, and Russia.

"But the stores are all closed, Tom. It's the middle of the night," he said, awakening and beginning to reason. Thinking feverishly, I had already anticipated his answer. "There's a twenty-four-hour supermarket on Lancaster Avenue," I countered eagerly.

My father was taken aback. There was indeed an open store in the area. Amazingly, he indulged me. He shook himself awake and said, "Okay, Tom. Wait here. I've got to get some clothes on, and then I'll be right back." I wasn't about to go anywhere. He got ready and took off in his car at 2:30 a.m.

I was wide awake and very hungry. My mind raced, anticipating what I would do once I felt better, imagining my qualifying exams at Columbia and how I would read all of the necessary texts and more. I lived through scenes of my professors and fellow students nodding to each other, oohing and aahing at my ideas . . . of learned audiences applauding as I entertained their questions . . . of governments calling me in as a consultant . . .

My father returned with a bag of fruit and a few other sundries for the house and found me ruminating over my acceptance speech for an endowed chair at Oxford. Thanking him did not even occur to me. Eagerly I grabbed a pear. Up close and real, it lost some of its charm. I put it back and chose one that was a bit more ripe—more likely to do the trick.

Greedily taking several bites, I packed both cheeks like a chipmunk and glanced at my father, who was busy putting away the other goods. Looking a little bleak under the fluorescent light, he was in his ingrained head-of-the-family post-shopping routine, even though it was three o'clock in the morning. The darkness outside the windows contrasted dramatically with the brightly lit kitchen. It was the wrong time to be doing this errand.

Suddenly my stomach turned and I ran into the nearby bathroom, throwing up the pear. I had not eaten since lunch on the airplane ten hours before. Something was clearly wrong with my digestion, not to mention my mind. After wiping my mouth with toilet paper, I retreated into the living room and resumed my curled-up posture. The fruit had not cured me.

My father reached a critical decision that night: I needed to be supervised by a psychiatrist again. Home care was not going to work and would wear him out very quickly. He did not mention the pear but climbed back into our improvised bed and tried to fall asleep.

I sat in the front seat of the Mazda the next day as my father and Tatiana took me to a local psychiatrist recommended by a friend of the family. Dr. Spalding was in his thirties, just a little older than I was, and had recently graduated from the University of Pennsylvania. He charged eighty-five dollars per fifteen minutes. My student insurance from Columbia would cover the first ten thousand dollars for mental disorders.

Dr. Spalding's waiting room was professional and cool, with wallpaper and carpeting, brand new furniture, and *People* magazine in the lobby. I sat in a single loveseat, not daring to lean backward lest my cast damage the soft leather or, worse, keep me from ever leaning forward again. I had no idea what to expect. Neither did Tatiana or my father.

CHAPTER 23

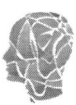

"What Seems to Be the Problem?"

The doctor invited us in and offered us comfortable seats. My hair was still standing on end, my chin still unshaven, though my father had persuaded me to change from weeks-old sweats into fresher clothing for the visit. Tatiana had painstakingly translated the medical report from the Soviet hospital into English for his benefit.

"So," began the doctor, smiling. "What seems to be the problem?"

My father burst into an account of the recent Moscow events, including my psychosis, the broken back, and his own rescue mission. The doctor interrupted him.

"What do you think is wrong with you?" he asked, turning to me.

"I was trying to understand the nature of social science, then I wanted to learn Greek and Chinese in the next few months . . . then everything went black," I said, not answering his question. "I was trying to escape the hospital to get back to Tatiana . . ." My voice trailed.

Grandiosity must have tipped him off. He quickly asked, "Who's the vice-president of the United States?"

It was 1991. "Well, let's see," I said, as though it were a question that deserved complex thought. "First we had Carter, and that would be Mondale, of course, and then we had Reagan, who had . . . now let's see, who did Reagan have . . . ? And then we had . . . who was it? I've been in Russia so long . . ." I had been in Russia two months, but I thought this was an elegant excuse. "I'm sorry, I've forgotten who is president right now. What was your question?"

The doctor made his diagnosis: manic depression. The way my mind was flitting from topic to topic was a dead giveaway. His next words were a relief to us all. At least someone seemed to be in control.

"I strongly suggest that you be hospitalized until we get your medications straightened out. The Russians had you on so many chemicals that it's going to take a few weeks, but we should have you patched up soon."

My father breathed a sigh of relief. "Thank you, Doctor Spalding. This is why we wanted to get Tom back to America." He didn't add that this was why he had fled from East Germany decades before, and why he had taken my rescue into his own hands earlier that summer. The limited opportunities communism offered were not good enough. Here I would get some real help. Better yet, the hospital was walking distance from home.

My treatment in Wilmington began with the gradual reduction of primitive antipsychotics from my system, letting what turned out to be the correct drug, lithium, take their place.

Along with their removal came familiar withdrawal symptoms: shaking, and an inability to keep down solid food. I survived on canned high-protein milkshakes. Then, as my personality began to reemerge, I would chat with the doctor on his visits.

I remember Dr. Spalding's first words to me upon my return to stability. I was lying in a sunny bedroom, overlooking a local graveyard, when he entered: strong, clean-shaven, and smiling. "Tom, I've got some good news and some bad news. The bad news is that you'll have to take lithium pills for the rest of your life."

My heart sank. No friend of medication, I took his words with a grain of salt, even though they were spoken very authoritatively. My father had set an example for me in the 1980s by overcoming his heart condition with diet and exercise alone. Now he was medication-free despite professional warnings.

"The good news is that if you stay on lithium, this sort of psychosis will never happen again. You have manic depression, and are one of the lucky eighty-five percent who respond well to the drug."

CHAPTER 24

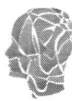

Flipping Eggs

I was released from the hospital at the end of the summer only weeks after my return to the US and took a semester off to live with my father and Tatiana at home, recovering my stamina and seeing the psychiatrist regularly.

I stabilized remarkably quickly, so well that I thought the whole episode might in fact have been a freak accident. The Soviet plaster cast was eventually replaced with a sleek under-the-shirt metal brace which, after a period of months, I was able to remove.

Maybe I did not actually need to take lithium in order to stay healthy. Two pink pills twice daily: they seemed so useless and unnecessary. How could mere pills keep someone from behaving like a wild animal? I often entertained the thought that my recovery had nothing to do with them.

Besides, along with those pills came the diagnosis: "mentally ill." I did not like that label. To me, the mentally ill were homeless or maybe psychopaths who needed to be locked up.

"I am not one of them," I thought. "I have never been suicidal. I have never been depressed. I'm just a graduate student who worked too hard. What happened to me," I reasoned unreasonably, "must have been a fluke."

I kept swallowing the little pink pills, though. I was terrified of what might happen if I didn't. The only side effect was that I needed to pee more often. Being so fond of walking everywhere, I developed "spots" around town: the library, the YMCA, the graveyard. The call of nature was stronger and more sudden than usual. But otherwise, I didn't notice that I was taking the drug.

During my semester at home, I tried to reevaluate my life. I wondered if this incident was fate's way of telling me to do something different with my time and energy. Maybe an academic career was not my path.

I looked in the classifieds for employment. It did not take long to find semi-skilled work near home.

"Dad, I just got a job as a short-order cook!"

My father, a gourmet chef, was delighted by this change in my intentions. He had seen graduate school turn me into a maniac. Now I could earn some straightforward cash by the hour, preparing food within walking distance of home.

But the deli was no French culinary school. I found sausage easy; omelets mystified me. Brought up on scrambled eggs, and with mania simmering beneath the surface of my medications, I kept fiddling with the egg mixture on the griddle instead of letting it sit to brown enough that I could fill and flip it.

I like to think that, with a degree from an Ivy League school, I could have learned omelets, but events at work got in the way of further training.

"Why did you use my receipts for scrap paper?" my boss asked, confronting me one day.

He kept his office door open, and inside it was about as neat as my room at home—chaotic. I had taken a phone message for him on a handy scrap. I always used extra computer paper for notes at home. At the time the word "finances" to me meant applications for grants and scholarships, not bookkeeping and the IRS. I had no idea the documents were vitally important for his business.

"Oh, I'm sorry," I said innocently. Usually that was enough to put me back in anyone's good graces.

The utter lack of emotion behind his words stung the most: "You're fired."

CHAPTER 25

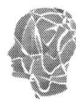

Back for Seconds

Fortunately I had a Plan B.

After my brush with the real world I was more convinced than ever of what I wanted to do: forget about working for peanuts and return to the shelter of academia. Out of respect for my father, I made a show of reading *What Color Is Your Parachute?* If any book could have convinced me that getting a job could be fun, that had to be the one. I figured I'd share my enthusiasm with my dad.

"You know, the number of clever approaches this book suggests for creating a job you love really bowls me over. I mean, it explains how you can convince employers that you're the only one who can fill a fascinating and vital position that doesn't even exist. And get hired to do what you love!"

The only problem was that it was all about that "four-letter word" my college buddy had sprung on me a few years before, and my feelings about work were no different now.

"How's your job search going, Thomas?" We were sitting at dinner. By now I was helping him chop and grate, slice and dice, and I could see he was encouraged by the amount of energy I was able to offer in the kitchen.

"Well, Dad, now that I'm back on my feet, I'm inspired to start accomplishing things again." I glanced over to assess his response. "I can see how soon I'll be able to use all the education I've been soaking up. I'm really looking forward to contributing to society." He was waiting for me to finish.

I figured I'd might as well break the news now. "I'm thinking that since I just have to finish my comprehensive exams and write my dissertation, I would be crazy to bail out before I get my degree." I couldn't meet his eye. I knew how much he wished I'd get real and climb out of the ivory tower.

He was silent for a moment. Many parents encourage their children in a particular career direction. He had always just wanted me to be content. "Okay, Tom," he finally said. "If that's what you think will make you happy." I suspect, looking back on it, that he thought graduate school would have the opposite effect on me, having been through it himself. But he must have thought I needed to discover this truth on my own.

I actually had considered finding a job that involved research and writing, since those were my favorite activities and by far the ones I did best, but in the end I returned to New York with Tatiana. I couldn't cut the umbilical cord to academia. We still had our apartment there. Tatiana returned to waitressing and planned to enter graduate school at Bryn Mawr on her own the following year.

In early 1992, I took two trial classes at Columbia. At least everything was paid for by a fellowship, not by my father and, of course, not by me.

Tatiana came with me but was emotionally scarred. She had seen me fall apart before her eyes and had been completely unable to do anything about it. Her helplessness frightened her the most. She had no family in this country besides mine to support her, and neither of my parents made her feel very welcome. My sister was living in Japan at the time.

"Tom, I am so scared that this could return at any moment." She began to cry. "I live with you like with a person who can suddenly turn into a beast. I do not know how to control you when you're like that." She began to cry more. "Tom, it's so terrifying to see you when you are insane. You're not the same person anymore. It's terrifying," she repeated.

We both returned to New York in January of 1992 in hopes that my illness was history, but she was aware on some level that it could surface at any time. Something inside her was broken. It wasn't my fault or hers. Our marriage was falling apart because of the illness.

"I can't believe you have to go down to Wilmington to see Doctor Spalding again already." Tatiana shook her head just a little as she frowned. "These days it seems like everything revolves around being sick."

"You want to come, too, and stay at my dad's? We could be back by tomorrow evening."

"You know I don't even like to be with your father anymore." Tatiana was still miffed that he had charged her rent.

"I just wish I could do something about my spine. It won't bend right anymore." I still hadn't gotten over my abrupt switch from perfect health to eternal convalescence in the course of a few months. My life, instead of blossoming as it had before my accident, seemed constrained.

Higher education is designed to generate curiosity. All the courses and lectures, all the seminars, all the office-hour chats have the same exciting purpose: inspiration. Students are confronted with these duties—tasks they would never encounter in the real world—to generate that special blend of love for a subject and desire to understand it. I took it one step further, though. I could not imagine any ambition besides more study.

I was every bit as curious as I had been before my psychosis, but there was a flip side: mania was still there, almost breaking through the surface, and it was making me rabid. I was intent on understanding everything at one go. It just wasn't realistic.

I refused to acknowledge that I was floundering, even to myself, and my thesis advisor in Russian politics preferred a hands-off approach. In other words, he was no help. The rear wheel of my mind's motorcycle was spinning on ice.

The obstacle of the qualifying exams still lay between me and my dissertation. At least my studies would have some direction before I was totally left on my own. Designed to force attention in many different directions at once, the tests leave students experts in their fields, ready to write an original thesis. These exams challenge one's capacity to read and simultaneously develop and express opinions on an enormous quantity of academic literature.

I joined a small study group after Tatiana and I moved back to New York. My only project for the spring of 1992 was to pass my exams, and my fellow students shared this goal. I assumed the leadership role I had become used to in my pre-manic life.

"So, what do you guys think that Clifford Geertz really meant in his article on ideology?" I pressed the group with an edge to my voice, leaning forward, choosing one of my own areas of interest.

"Hey, hey," one of the members joked, "watch out: this is what the comps are going to be like!" Everyone laughed. But I remained serious, singling out a Taiwanese student.

"Did you read him? Do you really think ideology is a cultural system, or is it more like propaganda?" I hammered him with technical vocabulary from my area of expertise. My heart was racing, as though I were a predatory bird ready for the kill.

"Say, guys, why don't we call it a night?" the host asked diplomatically.

CHAPTER 26

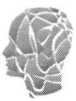

Tatiana's Turn

I passed my comprehensive exams by a narrow margin. They are called comprehensive for a reason—one is supposed to have read everything. I had overlooked an important book and, as a result, almost failed.

A little later, while we were snuggling, Tatiana said, "Now that you're done with your coursework, we're not really tied to New York anymore. It doesn't matter where you live when you're writing your thesis." That was true. I nodded for her to go on.

"I think I know what I'd like to do, Tom, since I didn't get to study Byzantine culture at Dumbarton Oaks. Can we do something for *me* now?" She could tell I was interested. "It's something a little more practical than Byzantine culture," she whispered.

"Anything!" I was delighted that she was taking initiative to move her life along. She had stood behind me as long as I had needed to study at Columbia and hadn't missed a beat. It was time for the next chapter.

"I could be a professor of Russian at some university. It would be a piece of cake!" I smiled at her very American phrase. "This is what we were talking about before! Doctor Hartmann and Doctor Hartmann in a nice intellectual community. It will work out after all! No more waitressing!"

That summer we moved to Bryn Mawr, Pennsylvania, where she could take advantage of the college's outstanding Russian department. I had studied there myself when I was first learning the language, and many of my professors were still around.

My advisor at Columbia for my PhD was that same hands-off, ineffective teacher who had failed to guide my studies before. I was having trouble centering in on a thesis topic, and it seemed he had nothing better to do than use his professorship at an Ivy League school as a platform for publishing books and articles about the Soviet Union.

"No interest in students!" I grumbled. I was getting nowhere and chose a vast topic almost at random: corruption in Russia.

We lived in an apartment building near the train station. As a graduate student, Tatiana enjoyed an allocated library carrel, a desk for her personal use. Since I was always most comfortable sprawled out in a library, I took over her spot, sagging its shelf with my own books. "You don't mind, do you?" When I was home dozing, sometimes she grabbed a moment in the carrel to work.

I commuted weekly to New York to give an undergraduate lecture. Occasionally we would visit my father in nearby Wilmington. An upscale video store just around the corner from our apartment building provided our only entertainment, and often, as in Manhattan, we would rent movies. Life was good.

I still lived with the routine of taking two pink lithium pills twice daily to stave off the Moscow horrors of 1991. Those times still visited me vividly in my dreams.

In February of 1993, Tatiana and I were hosting her mother on her annual visit to the States. Snow was predicted for the morning we were to drive Tatiana's mother to JFK for her flight back to Russia. "Doesn't look like snow at the moment," I commented over my oatmeal. Tatiana was preoccupied, picking at her fruit. Her mother washed a pan as she looked out the window. Hoping for affirmation of some sort, I tried again: "We shouldn't run into any problems on the road."

Tatiana's mother made a sound of agreement. In retrospect, I realize that Tatiana looked troubled, but as usual I was geared up and let it pass. I wish now that she had mentioned the nightmare that awoke her before dawn. In her dream, she had been struck by an oncoming truck.

CHAPTER 27

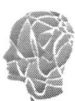

T-Boned by an Eighteen-Wheeler

It was, indeed, snowing heavily by the time we were on the New Jersey Turnpike, with slush accumulating on the highway faster than the tires of previous vehicles could clear it away. It has since occurred to me that the sensible thing to do would have been to drive slowly enough that the car wouldn't hydroplane over crushed ice, but I had never been in a major accident before and had a youthful sense of invulnerability. I talked with the two women, both of whom were in the back seat. "You were even eating a banana!" Tatiana later reminded me.

The going was bad. "I'm glad there's enough traffic to leave reliable tire wipes," I said in a chatty voice.

"Tire wipes? Tom, watch the road."

"Yeah, when you're bicycling in slush like this, the best thing is to ride in the clear path that the car in front of you leaves. The more cars there are on the road, the easier it is."

I was full of upbeat conversation as we approached Exit 12. That's where a separate truck lane peels off from the cars-only freeway.

"Why did we take the truck lane?"

"I figure it'll be easier. Those eighteen-wheelers leave heavy tracks, and there are a lot of them."

It didn't take me long to realize that the tire wipes were working against me.

I hadn't taken into account the narrower axle of the Mazda. The tires on the driver's side could roll unimpeded down one of the wipes. But unlike a bicycle, the car had two wheels underneath the passenger side.

The tires on the passenger side were now plowing through slush, dragging that side of the car back. I could have tried forging ahead with both wheels in the slush, but the Mazda did not have the momentum of the huge trucks tailgating me and whizzing by. There was no taking it slow anymore.

While I was driving with the driver's side tires in one of the wipes, the passenger side fell back so hard that the car turned itself into the lane, spun out of control and skidded to the left, eventually bouncing off the barrier that divided the eight lanes of traffic and coming to rest in the path of an oncoming truck, passenger side facing. We were all wearing seat belts and so far were uninjured.

The barrier stalled the car. As if in a dream, I tried to crank the engine as the truck approached. I was too panicked to think to shift. As I hunched over the steering wheel, laboring with the ignition, Tatiana's mother held her daughter's hand instinctively. Had Tatiana been sitting beside me in the passenger seat, she would have been crushed by the impact.

"Start the car! Turn the key!" Tatiana shouted from the back seat.

"What do you think I'm doing?" I yelled back, trying to remain calm. The eighteen-wheeler bore down on us, not attempting to swerve.

"Take the car out of gear," she advised calmly, perceiving the problem more clearly than I did.

But it was too late. In that instant, she relaxed. The oncoming truck smashed into the car and crushed the entire passenger side. The truck kept coming and the car, with us inside, hopped down the highway in front of it as the axles alternately compressed and released. Finally the momentum of the truck was spent.

Later, Tatiana clearly remembered the car's furious jolts and the feeling of her impending death. She made a conscious decision not to give up life. As for me, she saw my body flail around the driver's seat. I was strapped in only by the automatic over-the-shoulder belt.

Traffic backed up behind us. Knocked senseless but still moving, I waved my arms, lolled my head, and screamed nonsense. My mother-in-law, always one to care for her relatives, thought I was trying to get out of my seat belt to move more freely, and she remembered a Russian home remedy.

"Tatiana, my dear, Tom needs snow for his forehead so it won't swell. Open your door so you can get him some?" As she spoke, blood dripped from her mouth onto her white fur coat: her jaw had been broken by the impact.

Tatiana held her mother's mouth closed and told her to hold it. Adrenaline flowed into her system. Her heart was torn. She wanted to run away from all the horror she saw around her, but she felt a duty to stay and help as best she could.

She scrambled into the sleet, gathered a handful of snow, and came back to the wreck to hold it on my forehead. I was further confused by the new sensation and moved my arms even more violently, knocking away her ministration and screaming even more loudly.

Tatiana pushed her despair deeper into herself and held her mother's hand, stroking her face and weeping. Her mother looked back and smiled. "Don't cry, my dearest," she said, spilling more blood onto her coat as she spoke. "We're alive."

PART III

SMOTHERED BY DIAGNOSES

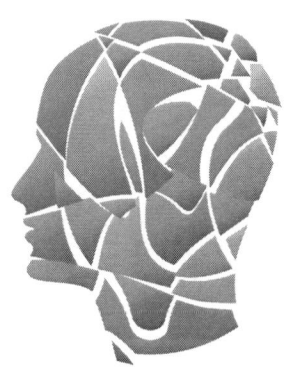

CHAPTER 28

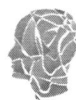

Two Times Lucky

"They asked me to come with them and 'identify Tom's body,'" Tatiana said to her mother, whose flight to Moscow had long since left without her. "They didn't even tell me first if he was alive or not!"

The two women had finally crossed paths again after several lonely hours in an emergency ward, where doctors had diagnosed Tatiana's mother with a broken back as well as the broken jaw that had been so easy to see. Tatiana had sat in the antiseptic lounge waiting for news of me while her mother was being examined, x-rayed, and wheeled upstairs.

"He is in a coma now, with some kind of brain swelling. Oh, Mamushka, maybe I shouldn't have stayed alive; I don't know if I can stand life like this! Do I even have a husband anymore? The manic depression was bad, but now . . ." She dissolved into tears against her mother's shoulder, trying to be careful about the broken back.

The coma lasted three days. Then a helicopter flew me on a stretcher to Graduate Hospital in Philadelphia.

During the helicopter ride, I was aware of chilly air against my torso for a while. Then I blacked out.

Subdued sounds awoke me. Tatiana was at my side and several friends were near the foot of the bed. Her presence made me feel safe and my heart reached for her. My friends smiled encouragingly. Gradually I was able to recognize some of them, but their features were blurry.

I had no idea that one of them had kept vigil with me for ten semi-comatose days to give Tatiana respite and time to study.

I looked at her questioningly. Was something going on? Scenes of our life together skipped across my consciousness. I exhaled, overwhelmed. "What . . . ?" I tried to speak, looking at Tatiana.

She smiled gently, stroking my hand. "Tom, it's so wonderful to hear you speak! Do you remember? We were in a terrible accident." She fell silent and I groped to get my mind around her words. Remember . . . speak . . . accident . . . ? I could feel her love for me, so I relaxed and didn't bother about the words. After a while she added, "It's lucky you're alive." Almost immediately I drifted off again, never having even acknowledged the other visitors.

The next morning Tatiana was by me again when I opened my eyes. On and off for most of the day she encouraged me to remember who I was and what had been happening in my life. I understood who she was, about both of our families, Bryn Mawr, our marriage, New York, my

PhD. Aha! My eyes lit up. Recognition poured into my mind like sunlight through an open window.

"When can I go back to Columbia?"

She was startled at the clarity of my question. I had greeted most of what she was telling me with nods and faraway looks. The tears in her eyes didn't mean anything to me, but I felt her tension and pain as if they had been an electric current between her body and mine.

The next day she greeted me at my bedside with some tantalizing news.

"Tom, the doctors say that the car accident may have gotten rid of your manic depression. Oh, I pray that it's true!"

I shared her enthusiasm. Even in my condition—trouble thinking, hazy vision, and difficulty expressing myself—I knew that manic depression was not something I wanted. The hated label "mentally ill" was one of the few things that stuck in my consciousness, just like my identity as a graduate student.

CHAPTER 29

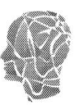

Looking in on Me

During my high school years, I had absorbed my father's doubts about the wisdom of doctors who had no better answer for childhood ailments than aspirin and antibiotics. His education, as well as his escape as a refugee from East Germany, had taught him how to think outside the box. He had sent me to the local homeopath for my sniffles and sneezes, inculcating a lifelong respect for this curiously effective sort of medicine.

When he had his heart attack in his mid-forties, though, he was subjected to modern techniques that he found primitive. While the whole thing shook me at the time in college, I largely forgot about the removal of plaque from my father's arteries ten years before. He didn't.

He had been awake and sitting half naked in a cold operating room as the surgeon made the incision in his leg. When the doctor blithely asked him to hold back the beating of his own blood by putting his thumb on his artery, it made a bad enough impression on him that he resolved never again to see the inside of a hospital if he could help it.

He applied his skepticism about conventional medicine to my predicament, too. When the doctors diagnosed my slow thinking as a brain injury, he thought he could help me find a cure, just as he had found one for himself against all medical odds. He knew firsthand that treating chronic illnesses is not the strong suit of standard medicine, and my recent experience in Moscow had confirmed his ideas. First, though, he needed to get me into a facility closer to home.

Once I was eating my own meals and remaining predictably conscious in Philadelphia, my father had me transferred to MossRehab, conveniently accessible by freeway from Wilmington.

I proved to be a disruptive patient there, and they didn't fool around. Before I knew it, someone had flipped me over and was jamming a shot into my rear. Within minutes male nurses wheeled me into Einstein Hospital's psychiatric ward and heaved me onto a bed. "Try to get some rest," one of them said.

It was still dark when I came to, uneasy and agitated. What was I doing in this new hospital? Heavily sedated, I tore off the sheets, slammed open my door, and made a clumsy beeline to the nurses' station. A strong male nurse was on duty.

"What," I yelled, "is going on here?" I did not have time to get out any more words. The muscular Irishman grabbed me in a half nelson and quickly walked me to the isolation chamber. The thick white door behind us cut off any noise from outside. He picked me up and bodily pinned me to a steel table in the middle of the room. With astonishing efficiency, he bound me hand and foot with straps. I struggled, and he tightened them.

"This is outrageous!" I shouted, but he left the room quickly. I remained with the sound of my own voice, without even an echo to accompany it. Wide awake, with no desire or ability to relax and fall asleep, I was aware of every passing minute.

I reflected on the incongruity of me, such an innocent soul, being tied to a table in isolation. In fact, head injury had worsened my manic depression, just the opposite of what the doctors had hoped. My psychiatric condition, earlier controlled by lithium, had blossomed into a case of blazing insomnia.

Only a month earlier, I had been peacefully visiting libraries, following academic pursuits. Now, even though I was not hallucinating, I was in isolation, and I felt it keenly.

"Someone!" I cried in the direction of the door. "I just want to see someone!" No use. "Just a face! Just look at me through the window!" I was crying. It seemed like torture. "I feel so alone in here! I'm wide awake and don't know what to do with myself!" I yelled at intervals for forty-five minutes.

"Please, someone!" My throat was growing hoarse. Suddenly I saw what looked like a nurse from the Indian subcontinent pass by my window. My heart leapt. "India!

Woman! I saw you! Motherhood! Sanskrit! Hindi! Deepak Chopra! Meditation! Yoga! Gandhi! Six-thousand-year-old culture! Ayurvedic medicine!" I free-associated, hoping to catch her attention. No use. Suddenly her face reappeared at the window. My heart melted as she looked in.

Outsiders are not allowed to say anything to patients in isolation. "Thank you," I said more quietly, "thank you so much." Human contact through a look. "Thank you. I'll be quiet now. Thank you." She continued to look at me. Tension seeped out of me into her serene eyes. She left. I was content to relax in my bonds for the night's remaining hours.

I spent the following day watching TV and eating meals with the rest of the patients, trying to make conversation. No one was really interested. Being with people who didn't even want to talk was baffling. I wondered if it was because of their insanity or, more likely, overmedication.

That night I still couldn't sleep. I was in the grips of mania. Again I leapt out of bed at two o'clock in the morning and dashed with my wobbly gait to the nurses' station to ask in loud tones what was going on. Again I was hastily accompanied to the isolation room. The big Irishman was getting used to pinning me down. He had already realized that I was weak and did not know how to fight well.

"Which one's your good arm?" he asked as he strapped me down. I moved my right. He left that strap a notch looser and put a urinal nearby. I spent another night waiting for the sun to come up. My Indian friend visited me at about four in the morning as I lay wide awake, staring at the small window in the door for any sign of humanity. She risked talking to me. "Concentrate on your breathing," she said. "You're doing fine." Though I could not apply her advice very consistently, at least I no longer felt alone.

I was given pills regularly, and soon they began to kick in. I was released from isolation and allowed to spend the night on the ward. Soon I began to sleep through until morning, but not without severe muscle twitches. Later I learned that this was a side effect.

My twitching caused me to doubt my doctors and their treatment plan. The newly brain damaged are notoriously muleheaded, and I was particularly so, given my family background of medical nonconformity. I began to secretly spit out my medicine, depriving myself of badly needed rest and risking the effects of withdrawal. Without my father, I don't know how I would ever have emerged from the hospital, caught as I was in a vicious cycle of noncompliance and forcible restraint.

"Dad," I whispered, checking to see if anyone was out in the hall to hear me, "they've put me on horse tranquilizers." Just seeing how calmly he was listening was reassuring. "There's no way I want to poison myself. I, um . . ." Now I whispered even more softly, and he brought his head nearer. "I . . . Dad, I've been spitting out those pills. They make my muscles twitch and I can't think."

On some level I had thought he would commend my good sense, but then again I could see how he might not approve. His response was measured and came down somewhere between those two possibilities. "Thomas, as long as you don't take your meds, you're going to end up in isolation, and as long as you're spending time in isolation, there's no way we can get you transferred out of this place. Ethically, they can't let you out on the street."

"Hmmm. I hadn't thought of it that way."

"It's pretty obvious you're never going to heal here. Let's put together a plan for getting out so we can get good treatment somewhere else."

That was okay with me, and I started swallowing the antipsychotics, even though the side effects reduced me to a quivering mess. I could not even hold my plastic fork to eat.

Within a few days my father had arranged for the chief of a local brain injury rehabilitation center to examine me to see if I could be admitted to his program. This, we thought, might at least get me out of the awful situation I was in.

In the meantime, I took matters into my own hands. I started spitting out my pills again by shoving them up between my upper gums and lip, lifting my tongue to show the nurse my "compliance," and then getting back to my room to flush the drug down the toilet.

CHAPTER 30

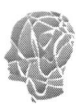

Withdrawal Pangs

Spitting out the pills was a terrible idea. In the course of a single day I began to go into withdrawal again, as serious as that of any drug addict. "At least I'm keeping down my food," I thought. My body was sweating profusely and shaking all over. Depriving myself of the addictive prescription meant I could barely get out of bed.

Had my withdrawal symptoms been more noticeable, the staff would probably have started giving me liquid medication. As it was, my agony seemed to escape their notice. I was stubborn about my noncompliance and after a few days the symptoms passed.

Not surprisingly, as the drugs left my system, I reverted to permanent insomnia. This time I managed to keep myself under better control so that even the doctors and nurses didn't remark. I was pleased I could pull it off. The only giveaway was my white-hot temper.

"Tom, I got you an interview with a doctor from the brain injury rehab place. Day after tomorrow, I will go over to talk to him and check it out. Tatiana and her mother are coming, too." I didn't tell my father that I was spitting out my pills again.

When the owner of the facility came to visit, I was lying in a bed in Philadelphia's Einstein Hospital. "How do you feel, Tom?" he asked.

My father stood beside him, smiling encouragingly. "I'd really like to get out of this mental hospital," I said guilelessly, with a noticeable lisp. I was accepted, but at this point I was not sleeping at all. My father had gotten me released from one hospital, but my underlying sickness remained.

My father, Tatiana, and her mother accompanied me to the rehab center. To leave the locked floor in the company of adults, wearing civilian clothes, made me feel as if I had somehow gotten well instantly—like passing from a dream into waking reality.

We had time to spare before our appointment, so we stopped at a street grocer beneath a set of train tracks in North Philadelphia. My father and I went to select some fresh food from the vendors while Tatiana waited in the car with her mother, who would return to Russia as soon as her back stabilized.

The crowd on the sidewalk was ethnically diverse, young and old. So soon after my release from the numbing routine of the mental ward, the vitality surrounding me was striking. My father negotiated the crowd and bought favorite fruit for Tatiana and me—plums and grapes. It was the first time I had been outside a hospital since the coma.

Standing on pavement felt unfamiliar, and I took special notice of food that was not wrapped in plastic. But I did not feel well. I no longer jerked in unexpected muscle contractions, but lack of sleep had left me dazed. I was as if in a trance. It took energy to concentrate. I was not cooking on all four burners but had no welcome sensation of tiredness. A pickpocket could have made off with my wallet or even my loose change and I wouldn't have noticed.

"It's no surprise you feel a little strange," my father agreed. "You're just emerging from a locked ward! But I think it will work out. Before long you'll be under the care of a famous psychiatrist."

At the time, mainstream Western medicine knew no way to facilitate recovery from head injury. This was shortly before the concept of the brain's plasticity became widely known. Conventional wisdom had it that some healing was possible during the first six months or, with luck, the first year after injury, but that brain cells were destroyed during trauma and could not be replaced.

The doctor had explained to me that the only variable in my supposed healing was the extent of the injury—that is, how many brain cells were left. Small injury, it was thought, was a loss that could be compensated for, at least partially. Big injury meant extensive loss and permanent disability.

The rehab center was located in a large apartment building on the edge of the city. The director met all of us in the lobby. We were to have an intake interview with the chief psychiatrist, Dr. Schwein. He was well published in the medical community and our collective hopes ran high.

At first my father was dazzled by the doctor's publication list. I was in no shape to remind him of the haughty advisor I had dealt with at Columbia, the one who, as he published one book after another, had proved that an impressive CV did not mean the author knew how to mentor students—a huge part of a professor's responsibilities.

CHAPTER 31

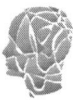

Dr. Schwein

Dr. Schwein certainly had the right appearance: a full beard and a white coat. He seated himself without speaking and faced our small family, leaning back and surveying me as if I were a specimen.

Tatiana's mother shivered in her chair. Later she told my father that even across the language barrier he gave off the most distant air she had ever encountered in a doctor. She was afraid for me to be in his care. It turns out that, on first take, she accurately "diagnosed" him.

"So, tell me your case history, Mister Hartmann," he said matter-of-factly, with a cool smile.

My father bristled. "Doctor Schwein," he said slowly in his German accent, "if you could do us the favor of calling Thomas by his first name . . ." My father's focus and intensity contrasted with the doctor's air of indifference. "There are two Mister Hartmanns in this room, and as for me, you can call me Doctor Hartmann." My father knew I was not quite "all there," but he was not going to let anyone lose sight of my humanity.

He and Tatiana were the ones who actually told the story from beginning to end: the Moscow incident, the recovery, the car accident, the hospitalizations. I started to say something every now and again, but each time thought better of it. On the few occasions the doctor turned my way, he seemed to look through me. To his credit, Dr. Schwein was at least following what they said, interjecting questions. As soon as they finished, he pronounced his recommendation, not missing a beat.

"Keep taking the same medication as in the hospital. We're going to start you on lithium."

Simple and clear. I did not like lithium much but remembered that it had kept me going in graduate school. The doctor, however, wanted to withdraw me very gradually from the Stelazine I had been flushing down the toilet. Should I admit that I hadn't been taking it? Hmmm.

It was unlikely that he would be as understanding as my father about noncompliance and my great dislike of the side effects. He might even tell me to get lost. Better to follow the intimidating doctor's orders and make a good first impression, even if it meant taking Stelazine again and experiencing side effects I hated.

Thus my father and I united against a physician who did not inspire honesty. It was hardly a great start for a doctor-patient relationship, but moving from the hospital in North Philly to an apartment building had to be an improvement. So what if I had to endure a little shaking, if it was the only thing between me and making a break with Einstein's mental hospital.

A few days later I was, no surprise, a mess of side effects again. Every night I went to bed and tried to keep the sheets over my convulsing body. Spring was just beginning, so there were birds outside. Over and over I waited eight hours for them to sing. My mornings were spent in rehab at a computer. The staff were trying to see if I could still think in complete paragraphs.

If I had actually had some sleep, I might have been able to write more coherently. As it was, the sleeplessness and grandiosity that were part of my psychiatric condition combined with the results of the head injury—insomnia, temper, and difficulty initiating anything besides eating—to create a ball of wax that no doctor would be able to unpack for decades. "Why don't you write something about yourself?" my therapists suggested.

"When I recover," began one of my paragraphs, "I would like to help Americans understand Russia better." I sat agonizing at the keyboard for the next half hour.

After my computer sessions, a matronly eye specialist helped diagnose my vision problems, a surprisingly common affliction for those with brain injury. Then I saw a psychologist. My afternoons and evenings were unscheduled. Following that, my night of torture would start again.

My temper flared regularly with the psychologist. It rankled me that anyone thought he had authority to tell me that I would never recover, especially somebody I considered a moron. Still basically a college kid, I always liked to question conventional wisdom, which in this case was Freud's.

My psychologist proudly displayed a framed embroidery of that father of modern psychiatry on his office wall. I wondered aloud why I belonged there, and then mused why he belonged there and not a more qualified psychologist, finally expressing my conviction that the brain injury center was a scam. I made a point of being a difficult client. Although I hated him for it, working with the psychologist eventually brought me around to the idea that I had a problem that needed treatment. Whether or not the center could help me was another question.

"No one should have to go through this." My father was having dinner with me in my apartment. "Look at your hands shaking. You're getting spaghetti all over yourself!"

"Dad, it's the drugs. I wouldn't have let them start me up if I hadn't believed the dose would come down." He nodded. "Don't you think I should just drop it again, like I did in the hospital? I'm sick of these side effects."

"Tom, I'll see what I can do. Hang on until tomorrow. We have to play by the doctor's plan; otherwise they might not let you stay here." At the time, staying there seemed like the best idea.

Next time he visited he had a pill cutter with him and a layman's drug reference manual. "This should start giving you relief tonight, Tom. We'll halve the dosage but keep you on it so the doctor doesn't think something is fishy."

Soon my muscle spasms began to reduce. As things leveled off, Tatiana joined me in the apartment at nights, but the connection between us just wasn't there. She was put off by my behavior and forced herself to be with me. My reality, meanwhile, had become relatively unsophisticated.

I had become a simple creature who laughed when he broke wind, yelled at her at the slightest provocation, and felt no compunction about spending her tiny graduate stipend on hour-long calls to college friends across the country.

I had not talked about ideas or subtleties, previously the substance of our relationship, since the accident. Nowadays my drugs, my doctors, and how I was feeling made up my only thoughts. She was no longer physically attracted to me. I was not the man she had married.

After about ten days, the psychiatrist scheduled another appointment at my father's urging. I was angry at the doctor for causing me so much discomfort. My father agreed that too many days of unsupervised suffering had passed before this cursory checkup. We both were present at the interview.

"You asshole!" I screamed when we met. "Look at me!" I held out my hand to demonstrate the shaking. My father signaled me a time-out. I yelled more about not sleeping at night. Dr. Schwein was not taken aback. I sensed, in fact, that he was smug. Giving strong emphasis to his words, he immediately recommended a stay in a mental hospital in Philadelphia for a few weeks.

I was caught off balance. His words hooked me, pinned me up against the wall, and left me dangling. Come to think of it, I had been ranting and raving. I looked speechlessly first at Dad, then back at the psychiatrist. My father excused us, saying we had to think about it.

"No way," he said to me on our way out. He was still smarting from seeing me in such misery at the mental hospital a few weeks before, to say nothing of Russia.

"But I think I want to go," I said, my own words astounding me. "I haven't slept a good night for weeks. There's something wrong with me. Maybe they can fix it there."

"Only if you think it's a good idea, Thomas. But I have my doubts," he said. I wasn't surprised that my father was ready to go along with hospitalization if I wanted it. The doctor's preferences were his secondary concern, even though I was certifiably insane. When he looked into my eyes, I met them with confidence. Even so, he hesitated. "The thing is, Thomas, once you're in a hospital, there's no getting out until they say so."

"It'll work out." I believed that somehow I would benefit from intensive treatment. Dr. Schwein's hospital had a good reputation. Moreover, the doctor himself was so well published.

CHAPTER 32

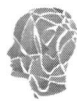

Humbled

The decor of the nurses' station reminded me of the thrift shops of Philadelphia's Main Line. Good-quality furniture, jumbled together without any sense of coherence, hinted that the ward itself was not a home but rather a way station for an unplanned assortment of passers-through.

"We're here for Dr. Schwein. He's expecting us."

The nurse put down her pen and took us to the director's office. For the first time in our encounters with him, the doctor was genuinely friendly. Now that I was firmly in the grasp of his institution, he seemed to relax. His demeanor made me suspicious: what kind of man only warms up when he has absolute power?

I was, however, shown to a neat, clean room, and was pleased to see there was no roommate. Since I didn't have anything to do until dinner, my father stayed a while, helping me get settled.

"I hate to leave you in this place," he said.

"Actually, it doesn't look that bad. Kind of reminds me of Russia." I laughed. "I mean, did you see that pay phone at the end of the hall? And at least the walls aren't entirely bare for once." I pointed to a framed print of an Impressionist painting, one of several, which hung directly outside my door. Turning back to him, I thought again of why I was there. "I can't believe it'll take long."

He agreed. "Soon those pills will be history. Well, good luck. I'll be visiting soon." A big hug.

I was left to my own devices until dinnertime, so I wandered the floor. After "lights out," I had a great deal of trouble sleeping and rose as soon as I could no longer force myself to stay in bed. At three in the morning I kept the night nurse company. This time I wasn't raising a ruckus. I tried to read the *Philadelphia Inquirer*, available on a coffee table.

Curiously, I was unable to read more than a few words before tiring. Instead my mind started drifting. I pictured my editor from my college days, when I had worked for the *Inquirer*. Later, while studying in Moscow, I had suggested some ideas to its foreign correspondent. I remembered a story that had made the front page and how important it made me feel.

Now I sat glumly, with blurry vision, not able to read, gradually becoming unpleasantly aware of how much had been taken away from me by the accident.

As I looked at the paper, remembering the heady feeling of seeing my ideas in print, I had a sudden flash of insight, something I am sure my psychologists had been trying to bring about: "My cockiness is not going to work for me anymore. People won't tolerate it now that I'm in this kind of condition."

Whether or not I liked it, that was how things were, and I just had to deal with it. I felt myself blush. There I sat, alone and distracted, across from a nurses' station, looking at words I could once have written myself, and my inability to read them humbled me.

This humility was the first good thing that came out of the accident. After all, several months before I had been caught up with my bicycle exchange as a minor actor in Gorbachev's perestroika and thought much more of myself than was realistic, especially at that point.

But even though my disability was slowly sinking in, nothing could convince me that my doctors knew how to help.

Action began to pick up in the morning as patients got up to have a smoke. Smoking, prohibited on the floor, was allowed on the six-foot-square platform of a fenced-in shaft that hung from the outside of the building. The area stank of urine, but it offered a straight view up Broad Street to the imposing tower of the Philadelphia Inquirer Building. The sight made me remember the day I had visited my editor there. I wanted to contact her.

Improbably, considering how little I had brought along from home, I had my telephone directory from when I was healthy, and I wasted no time calling from the pay phone.

"Sarah!" I mumbled in a heavily medicated voice. "I was just looking out the window of my hospital and thought of you."

I jumped right into the middle of a conversation without any introduction. Prior to the accident I might have asked if she had a moment to talk, but now thinking about others didn't occur to me. I must have made a strange impression, especially with my drugged lisp.

As I think back on it, I realize that she responded as best she could. "What happened to you, Tom?"

"Well, I got into a bad car accident, had a brain injury, and then had psychiatric complications." I was still compulsively honest. "I love to have visitors, Sarah." Heavy hint.

She was polite. "I'm sorry, I'm very busy now. Maybe later. Hope you're doing okay, Tom. Nice to hear from you."

I hung up with the sinking feeling that I had just made a bad impression. Sarah was no relative of mine, just a kind boss. Being completely open with everyone might not always be appropriate. Maybe work colleagues were not the best people to look to for empathy when crisis hit. I felt that I had just overused an old friendship.

"Who are my friends now, exactly?" I thought miserably. "Who still loves me despite my condition?" I recognized that feeling, so strong, so familiar: abandonment.

After I hung up the phone with Sarah, I picked it up again and dialed Tatiana. She was working on a paper.

"Tatiana," I said, "I feel lonely. When are you visiting again?" Demanding, needy, selfish, brain-injured me.

"Tom, I need to work for the next two weeks without interruption. I'm sorry, Tom. What's wrong?"

"I don't think I'm ever going to be the same person again." I paused. Then I said what was really on my mind. "Tatiana, do you remember, they interviewed me for the Rhodes scholarship?" There it was. I had said it. I wanted something to make me feel good about myself. Why not fall back on an old identity? Looking back was all I had at the time, but it was the beginning of a habit that would take me years to unlearn.

Watching my former life dissolve, I wondered if anyone at all would stand by me. At least I still had Tatiana. At least I had my father. At least I had the memory of the Rhodes scholarship interview.

"I remember, Tom." She spoke softly. No, I wasn't ever going to be the same person again. She did not tell me, "You'll be all right, Tom," or "Things will work out." The absence of those comforting words hurt me more than what she did say.

My medical diagnosis was "No Recovery." At the time, brain injury was considered a dead end. And a psychiatric disease, at best, would go into remission. I had not yet grappled with the full import of these ideas.

So Tatiana told me, "I remember, Tom." She was as hurt by the grim reality of the situation as I was. "I remember, Tom," she repeated. And then she began to cry.

"Tatiana, don't feel bad. I'm going to recover. Completely. Just you watch." She cried even more. Was it my disability *per se* that was so upsetting? Or that I was so much in denial about its severity? Maybe it hurt to see me banging myself against a brick wall in an effort to do the impossible.

"Work on your paper, Tatiana. Thanks for saying hello." I quickly hung up. Curiously, I felt better. By acknowledging the desolation of my situation, Tatiana had, in effect, cut out my work for me. I felt new determination to make the best effort at recovery that I could.

CHAPTER 33

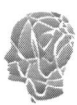

Just Being Friendly

Real trouble at the hospital began when my fellow patients elected me to be a gofer, the most responsible position a patient could hold. With this vote of confidence, I could go outside briefly to buy candy for other patients at a vendor near the hospital's entrance. Life on the ward was so circumscribed that even that small amount of freedom was an incentive for good behavior.

A patient from Israel was wheeled in on a stretcher with IVs. "Could you find me a Hebrew newspaper?" he asked surreptitiously. "Here's an extra dollar for you."

Newspapers, especially foreign ones, were not really within my purview, but I thought that solving a difficult problem for someone would win me extra credit with the staff, sort of like a complex homework assignment. After all, I knew the city well from being a student. "No problem!" I was itching to get outdoors for a noble cause.

I bought candy and cigarettes at the newsstand for the other inmates. Then I set off for the bookstore I knew was located near Rittenhouse Square, close to ten long city blocks from the hospital.

I'd been cooped up on the ward and the exercise felt good. I worked up a sweat as I covered ground to the bookshop. Still limping and sedated from the drugs—so much so that pedestrians cleared me a path and gave sympathetic looks—I congratulated myself as I made my way. "Boy, will they be impressed when they see my ingenuity in getting this newspaper. That guy is going to be so grateful!" I felt like a million dollars.

Then I thought of my college roommate and called him from a pay phone.

"Hey Mark! I busted out again!" I said, laughing. "Just like the big Indian in the *Cuckoo's Nest*!"

For some reason, Mark didn't think it was funny. "Where are you, Tom?"

"I'm on Walnut Street. Free as a bird."

"Hey, Tom, that's great, but, uh, I think in the book that was symbolism. Tom, I think you ought to get back to the ward. Tom? Are you still there, Tom? Can you hear me?"

"Symbolism," I repeated, letting the phone drop. I was heartbroken. I had thought he would come meet me. Desolate, I hung up the receiver. Back to Walnut Street and the beautiful weather. I found the bookshop and bought the only Hebrew newspaper they had on their foreign news rack. It cost me well over a dollar, but I thought I would absorb the cost for the sake of a new friendship.

When I had first heard about my new, privileged status on the ward, I found out that there was more to it than buying candy. If I proved responsible, I would be able to pay Tatiana a brief visit—actually leave the building for a few hours. I had not yet told her the news but was looking forward to a cup of tea or at least time on a park bench with her. Just the prospect of seeing her in a normal setting lifted my mood.

As I imagined how delighted we both would be, though, I remembered with a sinking feeling how turned off she had been at my lack of refinement since the head injury. I would make sure nothing about me disgusted her. Otherwise, it would be hard on her and on me. I resolved to shower the next morning and wash my hair. I even tried to think ahead about what to wear.

My fingernails, I noticed, were embarrassingly long after some weeks without care. The fact that it even occurred to me to think about grooming spoke volumes about my recovery, but I didn't know that at the time. I had been looking at outdoor gear in a shop window and went in to buy a small Swiss Army knife with the last of my money.

With the knife in my bag, I staggered the ten or so blocks back to the hospital. I entered the air-conditioned lobby, took the elevator up to my floor, and stepped blissfully onto the ward.

CHAPTER 34

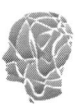

Locked Up Again

The schizophrenic on the hall greeted me. I liked her especially. She was an African-American, elderly and very friendly with large, drooping breasts, and she always wore pajamas and slippers as she walked the ward. She looked at me caringly. "I knew you'd come back, I just knew it," she said, caressing my arm.

"He's back!" screamed the male nurse on duty, grabbing the bag I had been carrying, which was full of stuff for the other patients. "You have a mandatory meeting with the head nurse in fifteen minutes!" he snapped, with a satisfied look. "And your pass to see your wife has been revoked!"

"What? Give me that!" I said, snatching the bag, fishing out the newspaper, and handing it back to him for a search. I had never liked this nurse. He was condescending to patients behind a thin veil of friendliness.

The Israeli was in the middle of the hall, laughing. I handed him the newspaper. "There you are. It was pretty tricky finding it." His face became angry as he glanced at the paper. "This is the wrong paper, you idiot! Give me my money back!" Now I was thoroughly demoralized, not even having been able to help someone. He was serious about the dollar, though, as if I had stolen it from him.

At the meeting, the nurse announced that I was being transferred to the locked ward the next working day. From the peak of privilege to the bottom of the hospital in twenty-four hours! I was furious. "I was doing him a favor!" I screamed. "You were out for over an hour and a half on a fifteen-minute pass," she said, just a trifle too evenly. "You will still have the same doctor downstairs."

The prospect chilled me. Back to a locked ward, and still with the hated Dr. Schwein. Shaking with disbelief, I choked on a lump in my throat. I could not understand why I was being treated so coldly after such generous conduct.

I limped back to my room and curled up miserably on the bed. I was more upset at being misunderstood than by the prospect of another locked ward. At this point, I felt I could survive anything.

Later that day, though, I began to think I couldn't stand it. I called Carter, my Haverford cycling friend, and asked him to help smuggle me out of the hospital. Everyone on the unlocked ward had "building privileges." That meant I could slip off the floor without attracting attention. He agreed to meet me in the lobby at a set time, and I prepared to leave.

Meanwhile, though, Carter began to wonder how to uphold our friendship without violating his own principles.

He called my dad for advice, and before long I was on the phone with my father.

"But, Dad, this place is nuts! They just acknowledged that I was a completely responsible person, I do something worthwhile, and then they get me on a technicality. They're really making a big deal out it, really playing dirty!" My father urged me to go along for the time being. At least, since Carter had begged out, no one had found out I was planning an escape.

The next day I was shuttled downstairs. The moment I walked onto the floor, I was assaulted by screams and loud music. A local station blared at full volume from the dining area—a nod to music therapy. I lay on my bed and scrambled to a corner, trying to feel the support of two walls as I contemplated my plight.

Occasionally the phone would ring outside, a loud purr over the screams. The noise was disorienting. Cries for help and wails alleging mistreatment mixed incongruously with the latest pop hits and advertisements for car dealers and sofas.

My first inspiration was to treat the horror and confusion of my surroundings as a game. During his first visit, my father played along. To boost my mood, he acted as if my transfer was not that serious; in return, I reassured him that it was educational for me to see what a "real" ward was like.

He folded my clothes into the heavy wooden drawers of my bureau. Our visit was short, and we parted with a hug.

Visiting hours were restricted to dinnertime. Trying to elevate my mood during the rest of the day, I interviewed patients, hoping to get to know them and learn what brought them to the ward. Unlike upstairs, talk here was not cheap. Women were suspicious and men were hostile. Were it not for the phone and regular visits of my father, my tiny capacity for self-sufficiency would have drowned.

One bright spot was when Carter came to visit, walking with me through the ward's doughnut-shaped hallway. He may not have smuggled me out, but he did prove his friendship.

"Being with you makes me feel like a normal person again," I said. "I mean, a person who functioned in the real world. Down here it's hard to remember that I used to be like that."

"You are a normal person, Tom," Carter said deliberately. His camaraderie did wonders temporarily, but it evaporated as soon as he left.

On his next visit, my father was dismayed by my turn of mood. Until recently, he had been expecting a release. Now my prognosis was unclear. The doctors, having watched me "almost escape the hospital," had put me in a place I could not leave. It was primitive and brutal logic.

I was in prison again. My father and I both vented our frustration at the system while he sat with me in the dining room. Soon it was time for him to go.

I made calls almost every moment that I felt lonely, using his calling card number. Telephone information gave me the numbers of old friends so that I could chat and lie about the stimulating pace of life on the ward. As I spoke, the noise all around me must have provided colorful accompaniment to my sedated lisp.

In my denial, I told them that I was thinking of forming a summer camp recovery island for those with mental illness. I avoided my feelings, which were too depressing to deal with. It became harder to find a sympathetic ear. Funding for the camp was a persistent problem.

Eventually I stopped kidding myself and started to feel desperate. I called home and said that I was tired of this game, that I didn't want to play anymore. At this point, I had been in the hospital for almost two weeks. The constant assault on my ears, more than anything else, was wearing me down. They wouldn't tell me when I could go.

This phone call wrenched my father's heart. I was facing up to my abysmal situation. What to do?

He talked to me about my friends, Tatiana, his plans to help me once I got out, how we would together find a way to beat the mental illness and brain injury rap. He talked to me as he always had, with respect, and it helped.

Sleep, though, was still a problem, and that was the real reason I was on the floor. My doctors were waiting for another symptom, something to help them make a diagnosis, so that they would know which medicines to give me. While this was better than the shock treatments in Russia, it was still brutal. Psychiatry is not an exact science.

Out of desperation I signed the patient release form found in all American mental hospitals by law, setting into action court proceedings. This document, a result of the patient rights movement, enables inmates to opt out of care. Finally, I would show Dr. Schwein who was boss.

CHAPTER 35

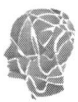

Inmates

By Dr. Schwein's orders, I was bound into a straitjacket for my court hearing. I suspect the extra precaution was only meant to humiliate me, but since I had just tried to bring a knife onto the ward, he had an excuse. Both of my arms were tied behind me around my rib cage, making it impossible to move them. The doctor did not bother to attend, sending his flunky to accompany me. My father came from Wilmington to the hearing in North Philadelphia to make sure I would be treated well.

The courtroom was crowded with plaintiffs, but I didn't see anyone else wearing a straitjacket. I hoped I didn't look criminally insane, with my dirty hair and disheveled clothes. I wiped the anger off my face as soon as I entered, replacing it with an innocent puppy look.

"What seems to be the problem?" the elderly judge asked me gently. My father looked back and forth between the judge and me, his concern evident. "The noise bothers me down there," I answered, holding still in my bonds. I had rehearsed a list of grievances, but none came to mind just then. The judge looked at the flunky. "Can we do something about the noise?"

I was happy to have finally asserted myself. "Sign another one of those forms," the flunky snarled as we left the courtroom, "and I'll make sure it's the last thing you ever sign." They herded me out of the room before I could do more than exchange triumphant looks with my father.

On the way back, the straitjacket didn't bother me as much. The respect and compassion the judge had offered raised my morale at the moment I most needed encouragement. Nothing was ever done about the noise, but it bothered me less now that I had made a statement.

* * *

By that time, I had a roommate. I was actually pretty lucky to be sharing my space with him, considering that most people on the ward were very obviously sick. Lionel was African-American, muscular, in his mid-forties, and friendly and open.

On my first evening back I had my usual difficulty sleeping, even though the radio was off and the screaming inmates were sedated. As I turned over in bed, my mind jumping from one thought to another, I heard a rhythmic sound coming from Lionel's side of the room. My mind cleared at once and my senses awakened.

"Lionel?" I whispered. Click, click. Before long he whispered back.

"Dry-skin lotion, man. They put it in your drawer."

So that was why they provided those little bottles of vanilla-scented lotion! "This hospital is okay after all," I said to myself, finding the lotion dispenser and getting back on the bed. "They understand about human needs!"

Sex, even solo, had always been an enjoyable activity, and after the manic depression began, my desire for stimulation had increased, sometimes to a degree Tatiana had not welcomed. Now that I was not being medicated and had been alone for days, I was feeling particularly randy. Lotion in hand, I went to.

Soon I was spent, and the stillness on Lionel's side of the room let me know he had satisfied himself, too. We both lay in easy silence for a while. Then Lionel started talking softly.

"Hardest thing about this place," he whispered, "is you're away from the people you love."

I thought of my dad, of Tatiana and her mother, and a longing for their company, the way it used to be, came across me like a wave.

"Yes, you're right," I agreed, genuinely heartbroken. We both sighed. After a little while he whispered again.

"That night nurse's going to shine her flashlight in here if she hears us talking. Then we'll catch it! Why don't you come over here so we can talk soft?"

Sounded good to me. I had been able to relax and experience the present moment while I was masturbating, but now my mind was racing again. Talking to Lionel would help me slow down, so I grabbed my boxers and went over and sat on the side of his bed, my long legs bent high at the knee, feet on the floor. He was still lying there naked and relaxed. His dreamy expression helped me unwind again. He spoke first.

"You got a girl? Married?" I told him about my beloved Tatiana, remembering the things I had most enjoyed about our relationship over the years. As I paused, he said, "I bet you two have a good time in bed." Actually, Lionel had been bringing every conversation around to sex since we had introduced ourselves. He sighed. "She's some fine woman, right?"

"Oh, yeah. You know, it's great when you're in love the way we are . . . so tender . . . I love it when she wakes me up in the middle of the night . . ."

"Mmmm. Sounds like you two have something beautiful going."

At that moment none of the post-accident horror was real for me. All I could remember was the sweetness Tatiana and I had experienced those first years before I became a brain-damaged, clumsy clown; before she started to find me a turnoff. Memories made me smile radiantly. "Mornings . . ." My voice trailed off and Lionel picked up.

"Hey, mornings are the best."

It didn't occur to me to ask about his loves, even though that was how he had started the conversation. Back then it never occurred to me to ask people about themselves.

My mind drifted happily through my memories of Tatiana. Lionel seemed lost in thought, too.

Then my mind was off again, flitting from idea to idea. So what was the story with Lionel? I had never whacked off with another guy in the room before. I wondered if maybe this was something normal guys do as teenagers and I had missed out on that kind of stuff because I hadn't had any close male friends in high school. Or maybe he had been in some other setting.

"Hey, Lionel, you ever been in the military? Or prison, or something?" That I could imagine.

He had pushed up onto one elbow as we were speaking, and now his body was facing me. He fixed me with his eyes. "Don't want to talk about it." He looked down briefly, then looked back. "You ever enjoy men?"

I was surprised he had said it. Not that it bothered me really. After all, my father had had a gay affair after the divorce when I was still in grade school, and his partner had been fine by me. Maybe I was a little taken aback because, truth be told, it is sort of a turn-on to masturbate with company. I guess it helps with the fantasy that you have a partner. I wasn't sure I wanted to confess that. I wasn't sure what he was after. Did he want me to say yes because he was gay and was looking for a partner? Did he want me to say no because he was straight and was nervous about me?

"Kneel down."

"Kneel down?" That snapped me out of my thought stream.

"Yeah, kneel down." Both of us had already satisfied ourselves not long before, so neither was aroused. I felt self-conscious all of a sudden, as straight as I am.

"What else?" I asked naïvely, as I complied.

"Just testing you." He laughed. "We ought to get some sleep. Get on back to your own bed." I skedaddled.

That was the beginning of a companionship I valued, my first real friendship as a patient since Dima in Moscow.

CHAPTER 36

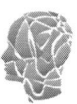

Tatiana's Visit

The receiver was dangling from the pay phone as I grabbed it, out of breath from dashing down the hall.

"Tatiana! You haven't forgotten about me! I had a good-behavior pass to see you, and then they put me in the locked ward, and then Dad said not to call you and . . ." The words tumbled out of my mouth. I hadn't given her a chance to speak. "Tatiana?"

"Hello, Tom."

"Tatiana, is there any way I can see you?"

"I was calling to tell you that I'll be driving through Philadelphia on my way back to Wilmington. I could stop by and visit. You are on the first floor now?"

"I've got to tell you about it. It was all so unfair." I was off again, but she cut in.

"I can be there in maybe forty-five minutes. Well, after I find parking, give me an hour."

I couldn't believe my good luck. It was as if dreaming of her the previous night had made her materialize. "See you then!" I hung up quickly and ran back down the hall. Lionel was in the day room as I came in, breathless. He glanced up, his face filling with a welcoming smile. I could hardly contain my excitement.

"Tatiana's coming to visit me in less than an hour! Today!"

He nodded encouragingly. "Hey, way to go, man." I loved him for caring about me. "Tell you what," he added, "I'll make sure I stay out here till you give me the go-ahead." He looked at me significantly.

"Really?"

"Go for it, man."

I ran back to tidy my room. Tatiana sometimes thought I was so far out of it that I wasn't even appealing, and I knew the clothes I had left on the floor would bother her. "Not today, though," I resolved. Lionel's bed was already neatly made. "Just like in the military," I thought as I smoothed out my own sheets, tidied my toothbrush in the bathroom, and even put the loose roll of toilet paper onto the roller built into the wall. When everything was ship-shape, I returned to the day room to wait. Before too long someone buzzed her onto the floor and steered her into the administrative office. I came bounding up.

"Tatiana!" Even I could see she was feeling hassled. I could have asked her what was happening in her life, if parking had been difficult. I could have asked if she had already had a long day. "I've missed you so much! I've been so lonely!" As always, I was only interested in talking about the biggest thing in my life: me. "Come on back. My room's not so bad." She nodded to the nurse politely as she left the office.

As we walked toward my room, I jokingly reminded her of our bicycling companion in the Baltics a few years back, the one who had offered to sleep in the bathroom to give us privacy. "Remember that? But you had set it up so we could stay with your friend?" With the suggestion from Lionel so fresh in my mind, it didn't occur to me that she might not be up for some "bedroom action."

"I'm afraid I can only stay for a small while, Tom." By now we were entering the room, and I stopped abruptly so that I was standing close to her. "I mean a really small while." She backed up a step and looked at me with what seemed like a warning in her eyes. I registered her sentiment, then remembered the sweet things that had sustained me the previous night when I talked with Lionel.

"Hey, Tatiana," I said softly, pushing the door closed, "how about . . ." She braced herself.

"Tom, you don't think I'm going to get into anything now, do you?" Was she glaring at me?

"Oh, I don't know," I said in my most charming style. "If you're not into it, maybe you could pay me a little attention . . . ?" Disbelief clouded her face.

"Tom, you're crazy!"

Her deft words pricked me. All I could do was echo them.

"Yeah, I *am* crazy, Tatiana. That's why I'm wearing pajamas in the middle of the day, locked on a hospital ward. Tatiana, you're my wife! Come on! Sometimes . . ." As I spoke, she exhaled sharply, popped her eyes at me, and left the room, slamming the door.

My spirit was crushed. Short visit! The impact of the door rang in my mind as I lay down on my bed and closed my eyes, rocking softly, trying to lull the abruptness of that brief scene out of my consciousness. I pictured Tatiana and me when we first knew each other in Moscow, our marriage that fall, then soothing images of life with our friends in New York. After maybe half an hour, Lionel tapped on the door and came in.

"She's beautiful," he said softly. "You're a lucky man." I didn't feel like a lucky man, so roundly rejected by my own wife.

"Hey, sometimes it all goes just fine, you know, and sometimes it doesn't." I stared at the wall as he continued. "There's ways of being crazy that women really like. I know that's true, myself, but there's certain things they just can't take. You be gentle, she'll be gentle." After a while he added, "Maybe she had a long day already."

Nothing could have made it all right. It was plain that the man who had replaced her interesting and facile husband was hard to tolerate. I could barely grasp that idea. I see now that on top of dealing with the new me, she was trying to process her loss. I couldn't offer her the compassion she needed in her grief.

I felt myself pulling away from my problems, locking my heart in a box the way I had when my mother rejected me. An hour before, I had been on top of the world. "I don't know, Lionel. I can't believe my marriage is on the rocks."

CHAPTER 37

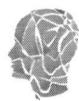

Isolation

For the next few nights Lionel and I both enjoyed ourselves solo, with the help of skin lotion. I had been miserable during the days but had kept myself from contacting Tatiana. It seemed as if one false move on my part might mark the end. My evening activities with Lionel helped me clear my mind. One night, though, just as I had gotten into it, I discovered that my lotion bottle was empty.

With the same naïveté that had led me to the bookshop on my ill-fated pass, I pulled on my boxers, sprang out of bed in the middle of the night, walked up to the nurses' station, and complained through the Plexiglas, "My hands are dry."

The nurse looked up at me from her book and pushed a button on her console. She told me to get some sleep. I took her response as an invitation to be more insistent. "No, I mean, my hands are *really* dry."

Suddenly the orderly appeared from a door behind the nurses' station.

"Tom, I want you to get some sleep." He handed me a hospital gown. "It's quieter in here." He led me firmly to the isolation room: an all-brick chamber with one small barred window and a bed in the middle. "Okay," I thought, "I can lie in here. Just don't lock the door." I obediently changed and lay down on the bed. I thought if I didn't resist, I might win a few points for compliance and would not be locked in. The orderly left and locked the inner door. Then the outer door. I whipped my head around to see what was happening. I began to yell.

"Hey, no fair!" Adrenaline pumped through my system at eleven o'clock at night. Barefoot and naked under my skimpy gown, I aimed a strong kick at the locked door. It responded with a solid thud. I lost balance, fell over, and felt the stab of pain from the blow and cursed loudly until the pain subsided. The hallway outside was empty and dark, but once I was convinced my foot wasn't broken, it occurred to me to reason loudly with the darkness, figuring someone with authority would hear how sane I was. I started in a conversational tone. "Let me out. I'm not supposed to be in here! Is anyone listening?"

The thick brick walls swallowed my voice. I tried again, a little louder. "Hey, I just wanted some lotion. Come on!" They were ignoring me, but I thought I could bring them around. "Hey, come on, let me out!" The lack of response was scary. What if I had to spend my life in here, locked away from civilization and unacknowledged even by the weirdo staff of the ward? That thought was enough to put an edge on my reasonable pleas, and soon I was shouting abuses. If I had realized that nothing I said would make even a slight difference, I might have quieted down. Instead, I got written up as "out of control."

The more I yelled, the more Dr. Schwein was convinced that he had made the right decision. I was losing sanity in isolation, and that was the safest place to lose it. I couldn't harm even myself there! The doctor, with his calculated coldness, had forced my psychosis to break through.

Although I had been relatively lucid when the orderly locked the door, I increasingly lost any sense of reality as time passed, partly because of the sensory deprivation an isolation cell offers—nothing to see, nothing to hear, nothing to occupy the mind—but partly because they had withdrawn medication. I was shaking again and hallucinating, imagining myself a zoo animal when I was grounded enough to be aware of my body.

I yelled for two days straight just to pass the time, alternating among Russian, German, French, and English. I counted in the various languages with the fervor of a camper singing "Ninety-nine bottles of beer . . ." hoping that a display of erudition would lighten my sentence. The staff were blasé about wild behavior. They merely took it as a cue to keep me in longer. Meanwhile, with no civilizing influence, it was too easy for me to act crazy, and I indulged myself with abandon.

The morning of my second day, the orderly visited me. "What are you willing to do to get out?" he asked. Looking back, I realize the staff must have been testing my capacity for reasoning: would I shut up in exchange for freedom?

"What if I hit you?" I asked innocently, convinced that I had been unjustly treated and feeling that somebody should be punished for inflicting such misery on me. My wimpy threat must have flagrantly failed the test. I was too angry about being locked up.

"It will be the last time you ever hit anybody," he said steadily, looking me straight in the eye. He locked the door again. Already in a routine, I screamed the entire day. I paced the room for hours. That night I peed against the brick wall of the chamber, feeling liberated by my utter seclusion and glad to be able to make some kind of statement. The nurses must have made a note of it and prolonged my stay.

On the morning of the third day, my throat was throbbing from yelling and the nurses were making regular checks. They served me breakfast and gave me medication. I ate eggs, toast, low-fat milk, and a debilitating dose of an antipsychotic, Serentil, in liquid form. I drank the milk slowly. It felt like cream, coating the raw inside of my larynx. Dr. Schwein and a medical student came in shortly thereafter.

Again I felt like his specimen, lying on the bed. He stroked his beard, crossed his arms in front of him, and rocked back and forth on his heels as he gazed down at me, smiling.

CHAPTER 38

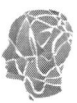

Paradigm Shift

"So, Mr. Hartmann, who is the vice-president of the United States?" I hated that smug, distant style of his. It was 1993. My mind reacted to the question like a tautly strung bow firing at a nearby target.

"Al Gore, of course," I snapped, turning my head away from his rocking figure. The doctor and his student left the room. I was exhausted by my yelling.

As the medication kicked in, I suddenly felt sleepy, and my strident shouts became whispers. At the same time, my senses began to come into focus. The silence of the room became palpable and I wrinkled my nose at the gamy smell of stale urine. It even occurred to me to clean it up with my own bed sheet.

I lay there forlorn, looking at my prison's door from the center of the room, my body feeling like a cement block. Around lunchtime, I heard a key jangling in the locks outside. My heart leapt. The inner door was left open and I got up unsteadily, then stumbled out.

"Free at last!" I managed to shout, despite the heavy medication. "Free—"

"Quiet down," said the nurse pointedly. I cringed and shut up, looked at her furtively, and staggered down the hall.

When I returned to my room, I found that Lionel had been gone for two days, released on good behavior. He had left behind a kind note: "Stay strong, brother." My clothes had been locked in a closet, and I had a new roommate, a quiet man, also African-American but darker and not as well built. My father, too, had left a note welcoming me back. I felt extremely tired and crashed onto the bed.

I was exhausted all hours of the day for the rest of my stay. I stumbled, sedated, to my meals and to the activities arranged for patients on the floor. I listened to the patient-staff "community meetings" in a daze. Overmedicated, I no longer had any trouble sleeping. My doctors had solved my case by turning me into a zombie.

I was soon released back to my familiar quarters upstairs. So that was good behavior—a drugged stupor.

Finally I was in the condition Dr. Schwein seemed to want, and, assured that I was debilitated, he decided I didn't need hospitalization any more. He couldn't break my spirit, so he drowned it so deep that not even I could find it through the swirl of new medication.

My father came to my room to take me back. Drowsy and moving slowly, I sat on my unmade bed and watched listlessly as he carefully packed my things from out of the closet.

"Where's Tatiana, Dad?" I said, my voice flat. "I was hoping maybe she would come." I had no idea what a burden my hospitalization had put on her.

"She said to tell you her work at Bryn Mawr is eating up all her time, what with writing papers, reading, and being a teaching assistant, too."

"Where's her mother?"

"She left about a week and a half ago."

"And I didn't even get to say good bye . . . I'm so out of touch with real life." The drugs took the edge off my regret, leaving only a blank awareness of my loss. Where was the depth of my feelings?

* * *

Back at the rehab center, the medication helped me sleep properly, but I was in a daze. Never fully awake and doubly clumsy because of the brain damage, I ended up only staring at walls. I spoke slowly and my eyes were glazed over, but I could still hold a conversation.

I had lost all respect for the staff there. The psychologist and I had a lasting enmity. When he tried to tell me, "You'll never be the same again," I pulled out my college vocabulary and spat, "Don't you understand what a paradigm shift is?" I was still lisping but rallied at the opportunity to argue.

He pursed his lips, putting on a patient expression. Well, okay, if this was my chance to grandstand, I would take it.

My dad, in touch with the scientific community throughout his career, had looked into brain recovery and discovered new thinking on the topic that had not yet made its way into institutions like this one.

I gave him a questioning glance, but he continued to look at me mockingly. I plowed ahead. "Hey, this is your field, not mine. Interesting how I know more than you do. Hell, they should hire me. You know, it's altogether likely that I will be one of the first people with manic depression and a brain injury to be completely cured." My face hardened as I saw him roll his eyes. "There's a huge sea-change taking place in medical science right now," I continued, my lips tight, "and you're completely clueless about it. You know, a *paradigm shift*? Conventional wisdom can change. I saw that firsthand in Russia. All of a sudden everybody realizes they were completely blind!"

"You sound a little manic to me, Tom," he said, emphasizing his words by raising his eyebrows quickly. But I was serious.

"I'm not saying it won't take a lot of work, but think big for once." I tried to catch his eye. "That's the only way to make a difference in this world. I'm ready to devote myself to healing completely from this injury, and here you are telling me I should go make baskets somewhere. You're the basket case!" How ridiculous he looked, sitting there under his Freud embroidery.

I hadn't been this worked up in a while. Somehow I had pushed myself past the point of exhaustion and was flying on automatic. It felt good to be fully charged, and I was glad to put him in his place. It infuriated me that he didn't meet me on my own ground, as if he hadn't listened to the substance of what I had said.

"Statistics show that healing stops after the first six months," he said, smiling. His satisfaction irked me.

"What about statistical outliers?" I could still talk like a graduate student, even if I couldn't think like one.

"Don't you think you're being a little grandiose? Grandiosity is a symptom of manic depression," he said, smiling again.

My fury boiled. "F*ck you, Frank!" Such violent anger did indeed demonstrate that I was not over my injury yet. "You guys here are only interested in making money off brain-injured people and keeping them sick."

I stomped out of the psychologist's office. Word had it around the center that the director drove a white Porsche and saved a black Porsche for the cooler months. He was no fool, having become rich at the expense of the brain-damaged clients the center exploited. My father caught wind of the center's greed when the insurance bills came in, reinforcing the idea in my mind that the staff had a vested interest in keeping us all there as long as possible.

Arguing with the psychologist had kindled low-grade manic energy in me, and I wanted to keep talking. My recent memory of almost getting one of the highest honors in the country supported my illusions. During my father's next visit, I let him know of my frustrations.

"Cutting off hope of getting well means essentially giving up on thinking altogether," I said to him, "and thinking feels good. It's what I like about myself." He knew it was true. "Besides"—I sprawled on my dinette chair—"what does Western medicine know? They can probably fix head injuries in China and India. I just need to research it, and if anyone can research something, I'm the one.

"I want to leave," I concluded.

"You're not better yet, you know," he said.

"I know, but they can't help me here."

He sighed in agreement. Within the week I had checked out and was free to solve my problems without professional guidance.

PART IV

TREATMENT AT HOME

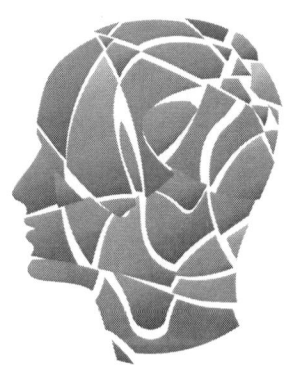

CHAPTER 39

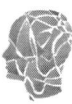

"Learn a Language"

At our kitchen table, my dad pulled out his phone directory. "Should I make the appointment with Charles, or can you handle that?" Charles was his acupuncturist of long standing.

"I can, no problem." I knew my father would take it as a good sign if I handled my own business. "The more responsibilities I take, the better I'll feel." My father nodded approvingly and handed me the phone, pointing to the number.

I had been fascinated when I heard about Charles' out-of-the-way carriage house and was longing to check it out. The story my dad told me had given it mystique: after Tibetan monks saw it in a vision, Charles "knew it had to be," managed to locate it, and moved in shortly thereafter.

My dad was perhaps not the only DuPont scientist who thought outside the medical box, but he was among those who lived their ideas out most fully. I grew up taking his example for granted.

After my parents split up in the early 1970s, he had begun to explore Eastern thought and practices and had incorporated a lot of what he learned into his lifestyle. The elegance of some of these approaches, like preventing disease through simple yoga movements, fit well with his frugality—a common German trait that was especially pronounced in him because of his refugee background.

It was not hard for my mother to cast frugality as cheapness, something she had identified in him long before and spoke of bitterly. As I grew up, instead of admiring his remarkable ability to improvise solutions to health problems, I would roll my eyes at his preference for Eastern solutions and say, "Dad's on his psychic kick again."

Still he persisted in learning all of the classical Tai Chi positions and doing yoga and meditation. He also became acquainted with a circle of Eastern immigrants who practiced medical traditions most people in America hadn't even heard of. He gave such original thought to the "mind-body connection" that he eventually opened a type of physical therapy business himself and called it The Mind-Body Practice.

Until that point, I hadn't paid much attention, but now that I was so sick myself, I was ready to reap the benefits of his experimentation. I trusted his judgment as he steered me to healers he knew. It would be my first acupuncture session, but given his example, I was not particularly afraid.

By this time, Charles had answered the phone. "Why don't you two come over right away, and I'll see what I can do," he said. "It's well known in China that the right treatment immediately after a brain injury can alleviate many symptoms." It wasn't exactly immediately after the accident at this point, but the sooner the better.

His carriage house was clean, with high ceilings and large windows looking out on acres of trees. The place exuded aristocratic comfort. I lay face down on a wooden cot covered by a sheet. With quick authority, Charles tapped short needles into various spots on my head and back. None of them hit a nerve or drew blood. Soon I could hear him talking to my father in the next room.

After five minutes, I was already impatient. There was nothing to do except lie there. I started to wiggle my arms but found that even the slightest movement jarred the needles enough to cause an unpleasant stabbing. I tried not to fidget as I thought about how nice it would be to check out Charles' fridge. He returned just as I was preparing to call out for him.

"Did you forget about me in here, Charles?" I asked playfully.

"Nope. I was only gone fifteen minutes or so."

I saw him regularly for a few more weeks, but my father, wanting faster results, sought out a Chinese herbalist on Charles' recommendation.

One morning Tatiana awoke to look at me with a piercing gaze. "What are you thinking about, Tom?" she asked, evidently trying to understand my disability sympathetically.

"Nothing," I answered as I turned my head, my blank blue eyes looking straight into hers. My mind really was vacant. She threw off the covers in disgust.

"If I were in your position, I'd learn a language," she said, misinterpreting what was actually my relatively precise description of brain damage and overmedication—a blank mind—as laziness. Being the daughter of a philology professor, she knew five languages and was familiar with what fun it was to learn them. Lazy people need to be inspired with an idea, a challenge. But I was not exactly lazy. I hadn't let my mind's engine disengage; rather, it had stalled entirely, sort of like the car in that fateful snowstorm.

Lazy. She wrapped herself in a towel and stepped downstairs to the shower. She had a lot of work to do today. She was earning a stipend for both of us.

CHAPTER 40

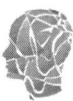

Shanghaied

"Breakfast is ready, Thomas!" came the enthusiastic call from my father downstairs. Food! I threw off the covers, put on some dirty clothes, and made my way down, missing my footing on two steps but managing not to fall. I was still suffering from a serious limp.

I burst into the kitchen. "Pancakes! On a weekday!" I didn't need to say "thank you" in words; the light in my eyes said it all.

My dad smiled. "Celebration of your return to civilization!"

I heaved myself into one of the sturdy kitchen chairs, so hard that it bounced to absorb the impact. I pulled up to the table before the steaming pancakes and reached for the small bottle of syrup, emptying it onto my plate. "Boy, that looks good!" I said, grinning as I cut off an oversized mouthful and stuffed it in. "We hardly ever have maple syrup in this house, and this is the real stuff!"

As a matter of fact, the syrup had been a rare commodity. My father raised his eyebrows. Tatiana, shocked at my poor manners, looked at me in disgust while he tried to engage me in conversation to get me to slow down.

"Like the syrup, Thomas?" I nodded my head vigorously and smiled broadly, small pieces of pancake sticking out. Tatiana threw down her napkin and got up to wash her dishes. I wiped my mouth with my hand and continued to devour the food.

Her life was becoming an exercise in damage control. One afternoon in October I came home to our attic apartment and looked around at our miserable living conditions—no plants, no computer; just a small file cabinet, a desk, a bookshelf, and a futon bed.

Suddenly I was seized by the idea of giving the place a thorough cleaning, so that it would reflect my inner emptiness and I would feel more at home. I started by dumping our bookshelf into the large plastic trash bin we used instead of a wastepaper basket. Satisfied, I made my way downstairs.

When Tatiana came home, I had already forgotten about my earlier wholesale purge. I was sitting at the kitchen table when she entered, furious. "Why did you throw out all of our books, Tom?" It briefly crossed my mind that living with others involved accommodating them, now that I was no longer hospitalized.

"I wanted to clean up," I said sheepishly. Now, some twenty years later, I realize that this must have been one of the key moments in the erosion of our marriage. Brain trauma made me like a selfish child in a grown-up body. It was hard for Tatiana to get used to.

As for me, besides brief moments of self-awareness, I never perceived how my muleheadedness was wearing out my father and Tatiana. Nor did I pay much attention to how therapies might interact or conflict with each other. As I saw it, I would bring about my own healing and everyone should bow to my needs. I would improvise a recovery, just as I had put together the bike trip.

This time there was no Plan B. One night I overheard Tatiana and my father talking.

"Tatiana, I just have to take it on faith," he was saying. "At this point, all I can do is recommend people I trust to him. We've already seen what conventional medicine has to offer, and I'm not impressed. It's turned him into a zombie, and on top of that, he's miserable."

"Miserable? Miserable! I am, too. Aren't you? He doesn't understand that there are some things he just can't do. After all, how much improvement is really possible?" I was standing out in the hall, feeling I shouldn't be listening. She continued. "I don't have the heart to tell him how hopeless it all seems to me."

"Well, at least I know some good healers. It all comes back to what I told that man in the airport when we were leaving Russia: 'This is my son! What would you do?' I'm afraid of phonies, too, but I want the best for him. After all, the insurance money would be gone by now had he stayed in rehab."

"And there's no telling him no." They both sighed. I turned to quietly make my way upstairs.

* * *

The herbalist Charles had recommended was also located in Wilmington's western suburbs. Fortunately, a real doctor from China was visiting, one of the few who had survived the Cultural Revolution. He was a specialist in acupressure and herbal medicine and was working for the local Chinese entrepreneurs who ran the shop selling herbs. By this time, my one-track mind was focused on how to heal.

Bald, hunched, and smiling, the acupressurist introduced himself with a handshake and told me to lie down on his table, a bamboo cot. The office smelled of dried leaves, like a day in autumn. Chinese art decorated the walls. A cat made of silk gazed out at me as I turned to look at the doctor's paper-strewn desk.

One trick of Chinese medicine is to insert acupuncture needles into the ear to take away the desire for nicotine. On the strength of word of mouth, smokers had flocked there to be cured. The shop had even gotten local press coverage and subsequently raised its rates. A shiny new car graced the entrance.

It was evident to the doctor that I had come with a complaint more serious than smoking. The shopkeepers had explained my condition to him in Chinese, then left me to his devices. I lay on his treatment table. I was not afraid that he would do any harm, since I had inherited a respect for the ancient Chinese tradition of medicine through Tatiana's father as well as my own. Not only that, but the doctor was genuinely friendly.

He seemed to know the herbs for everything. Colds? Not a problem. Was the sex life a little difficult on heavy medication? He had the answer for that, too. What's more astounding, it all seemed to work.

His profession involved pressing hard with his fingers at certain points on the body. He worked over my legs, head, and neck, seeming to take it all very seriously. I enjoyed thinking that he was taking on a tough case. While he treated me, he related how during the Cultural Revolution he had wandered from village to village in China with only his hands as his medicine bag.

After the treatment, the entrepreneurs gave me packages of dried leaves to cook later that evening. I was to drink the resulting mixture like a strong tea, and to add two raw eggs to the potion. Eggs are made of protein, as is the brain.

Feed the brain, and maybe it heals. Maybe.

Later that evening I followed their directions exactly. The medicine tasted awful, the only good part being the eggs. I was ready to do the treatment until I saw improvement, though. I was desperate—the perfect candidate for quackery.

After a week of treatment, my father drove me to the herbal shop once again. We were quiet in the car. Classical music played. His car, new after the accident, was tidy.

I greeted the smiling doctor in his improvised office. "Any improvement?" he asked. He expected immediate results.

"Well," I said, "not really, but maybe I need to try some more." I wanted to give him the benefit of the doubt. He was my only hope. If he was a quack, I was about to be taken.

CHAPTER 41

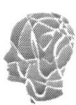

Monkey Mind

"Ah, I will try something I learned in Shanghai. We have research institute. Inject blood into rat's brain. Give them herbs. After herbs, no blood in brain. We tried on one girl who got hit with baseball bat on head. Major hematoma. Recovered completely." He smiled and nodded his head. He reminded me of Yoda in the *Star Wars* trilogy. It sounded too good to be true. The doctor padded off to call for the shop owners in Chinese.

I had told the herbalist that my head trauma had been a closed one, the kind that involves internal bleeding and damages the brain with pressure from the blood. It sounded to me as if the doctor was right on target. This approach to the injury seemed more elegant than the one often used in cases like mine—drilling a hole in the skull to let the blood out.

I was not surprised that the Chinese had a remedy that Western doctors were not using. Language and culture, to say nothing of politics, are serious barriers for the medical profession. Also, Western medicine likes to isolate active ingredients, test them, and produce them artificially, something not easy to do with remedies like this one that supposedly work synergistically.

The doctor shuffled back in and handed me a new package of leaves to boil. "You try," he said. "You see." Doctors in China aim to please. Traditionally, they were paid only if the patient recovered. I left the office with renewed hope. Drinking eggs and bad-tasting tea for the rest of my life was an unpleasant prospect, but I had talked myself into it over the course of the past week.

The new decoction tasted no different. I had been told to add raw eggs again. Immediately upon arriving home, I took it.

People with healthy brains are entertained, bothered, inspired, or nonplussed by a never-ending stream of thoughts. A sharp mind is aware of an interesting idea when it surfaces from the unconscious and marks it carefully before it is lost again in the babble, maybe sharing it with someone or writing it down.

My mind, though, did not work that efficiently. No new and interesting thoughts had occurred to me since the car accident.

I thought exclusively about what I used to know. I got bored as soon as there was nothing to do or eat. The dual problem of blurry vision and a stalling brain kept me from reading. Hours of agonizing free time filled my schedule.

My longing for sexual stimulation preoccupied me, but I felt I had to restrain myself with Tatiana. Mostly I waited for her to appear, for a meal to manifest, or for a trip to the doctor. If my father and I had never identified any new possibilities, it might have made sense to stay at rehab and train for less demanding work, not that I would have had the patience to do it.

That fall, in 1993, I looked forward to Sundays because I could take a long walk and go to the local Quaker meeting. To me it was like being communally bored for an hour, and that, in my view, was better than being bored alone for any amount of time. One day, however, the hour of silence that characterized the worship had new appeal for me: it became an opportunity to think.

On the way home from a meeting shortly after my second Chinese treatment, I walked through one of the more depressed areas of Wilmington. Suddenly a thought entered my mind: why not establish a house-by-house urban renewal project? It would inspire high school and college students to public service and rehabilitate homes at the same time. After all, I had been Mr. Volunteer Work in college. I began to wonder whom I could approach about the idea. Somebody in the city government? In the neighborhood?

Thinking in terms of interesting projects had a welcome familiarity. How expansive I suddenly felt, thinking about something other than myself. I saw the area with new eyes as I envisioned the improvements that could be brought about on that blighted street. This was the me I knew!

For the first time in the better part of a year, I recognized the idealist in me. I was elated. I limped home with a pronounced bounce to each step.

Only when recalling the episode that evening did it even occur to me that the Chinese potion might have been responsible for my sudden improvement. Single-mindedly, I resolved to keep drinking it until I was sure of a total cure. The change really had been remarkable, and since I was expecting a miracle, now I had something to point to. I had no grasp of the medical implications of "blood in brain," but I could think of no reason not to be completely optimistic.

I came home and announced to my father that I was feeling like myself.

CHAPTER 42

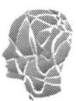

Salt for Sale

"Great, Thomas," he said, without much excitement. He was fixing the kitchen drain and did not turn to look at me. After my frequent affirmations of certain healing, beginning with the pear, he was skeptical of claims about major changes in my condition.

"Since you're feeling so fine, how about making dinner tonight?" He ran the household alone and Tatiana was at graduate school until eight or nine in the evening. My helping with food preparation would be very welcome. He was also tossing out a challenge. After living with me briefly, my father had realized that love and pampering would not cure me of my injury. He had begun to lay down rules for me to follow and household chores for me to do.

"Sure!" I said, eager to demonstrate my newfound health. I grabbed my favorite cookbook from the shelf. Before the accident, I had been able to improvise meals based on what was in the refrigerator. Its contents now held no interest for me. Instructions were easier to follow.

"One half teaspoon salt," I read. I checked the kitchen's salt supply. The empty shaker stood between the oil and a large bottle of soy sauce in the cabinet above the stove. My food preparation efforts came to a crashing halt. "Dad, I'll be right back," I called. He was now upstairs. I was making an emergency run for an ingredient. Good cooks do that all the time. I had seen him do it.

I selected the store's generic brand from the variety of cylindrical containers without actually checking the price. From my college days I remembered that salt was cheap and figured price shouldn't matter that much. The checkout line was slow. I returned home fifteen minutes later with my prize.

My father was already cutting vegetables for the meal. "Where were you?" he asked, somewhat annoyed that he had needed to jump in to help me fix the meal. He had, after all, been busy trying to repair the sink.

"We were out of salt, Dad," I said, in a tone of voice that implied that I had taken care of an important chore.

"Salt is on the shopping list, Thomas. You know we'll have some the next time I go to the store. Did you at least take the shopping list when you went?"

"No," I said, feeling my balloon deflate.

"Well, we have plenty of soy sauce. Why didn't you substitute with soy sauce? You know this cookbook likes to use salt instead of soy sauce, don't you? You're the one who told me that."

My feeling of sudden recovery was now completely gone. His mention of my competence before the accident seemed unfair. The comparison itself was a compliment, but he was setting the bar for my recovery awfully high. I realized that I was still sick.

"Anyway, did you get the cheapest salt?" I remembered that I hadn't checked. The location of injury in my brain had impacted precision.

"Yes," I lied. I couldn't face too many blunders at once.

"Well, that's good," he said, and gave me a hug with one arm. "Let's finish cutting these vegetables. I'm hungry."

My experience with the Chinese doctor did, however, give me the conviction that turning to alternative medicine is effective and that brain injury is treatable. I remembered the Philadelphia rehab center and felt sorry for its clients. I made a special trip there to show off my progress.

CHAPTER 43

Calling the Professor

Between patients the psychologist saw me for a moment. "Astragalus. Big capsules with herbs in them," I said proudly. I took out my afternoon dose to show him and threw it down my throat. "You take those without water?" he asked, amused. If he thought that I had actually found something effective, he pretended not to notice.

"Can those cure hemorrhoids? I've got terrible hemorrhoids." He laughed.

"Yeah, I'll bet . . ." I thought I'd better stop there, so I stood up. So much for changing conventional opinion. Maybe he was just getting back at me for giving him such a hard time.

As I walked out, I came to a decision: no more clowning around trying to convince closed-minded people. From here on out, I would concentrate on getting myself well first, and if anyone wanted to come along for the ride, they were welcome.

I began to try any medical tradition if it offered some hope of recovery. I was not afraid of quackery. The worst my experimentation could do, or so I thought, was not work.

I couldn't believe any alternative treatment could do as much harm as the antipsychotic medication I was still taking. Those pills continued to make me lethargic and clumsy, and when I spoke, they made the words come out with a strained inflection. I would never have noticed the difference—it's hard to assess the sound of one's own voice—had my father not, in hopes of convincing me to "get real" about my progress, told me to listen carefully to my answering machine message, recorded before my head injury. On it, I sounded crisp and professional, a humiliating contrast to my new voice, so devoid of subtlety or presence.

I added monthly acupuncture visits to my routine of sleeping, eating, lying in bed, and seeing Dr. Spalding, the same psychiatrist who had pulled me out of mania after Moscow. It was becoming a full-time job for me to get better.

Feeling particularly bold one evening, imagining that I had recovered enough and with great nostalgia for my former self, I placed a call to a favorite professor at Columbia. I still had his home number in my daily planner.

"Hello?" answered the kind, familiar, distracted voice of the man who had taught me in my healthy years. Classical music played softly in the background. It was nine o'clock in the evening, on the verge of being an impolite time to call.

"Professor Bernstein? This is Tom Hartmann. If you remember, we met briefly last year at a café on Broadway." I still sounded heavily medicated.

"Yes, Tom, I remember," he said kindly. "I'm sorry to hear about your accident. Please excuse the music in the background; my back goes out now and again. I'm lying on the floor, listening."

"I'm sorry, Professor Bernstein." I did not make conversation. I jumped right into my question. "I wanted to ask you about Max Weber. I find his *Sociology of Religion* very difficult to read. Is there any alternative?" Approaching a professor during office hours or class is standard procedure; phoning his home at a late hour pushed the boundary of decorum.

"You know, Tom, other authors have taken parts of that essay and done things with it, but there's really no alternative to digging into the original material." He went on to name the authors, their works, their ideas. In short, he offered me a private, off-the-cuff lecture.

I heard him out, thanked him, wished him a good night, and hung up.

"Who was that, Tom?" asked Tatiana, freshly upstairs from watching TV.

"Professor Bernstein," I answered sheepishly, knowing she would object. My interest in Weber, the subject of intense reading just before the accident, was a sign of my disease and my inability to adjust and get on with life, not an indicator of recovery. But I always answered her truthfully, that being the safest way to avoid an argument.

"Tom," she asked, immediately waxing angry, "why were you talking with Professor Bernstein on the phone on a weeknight past nine o'clock?"

"I had a question," I said, even more embarrassed. I felt like a child being disciplined.

"Tom, my stepfather occasionally gets calls with 'questions' from mental institutions. You know, Tom, he always answers them kindly, and to the point. Do you know the looks we exchange at the table after those calls? He gives them an answer because he feels sorry for them, Tom. Do you want Professor Bernstein to answer you because he feels sorry for you? Do you want him to respect you or not?" Seeing that I wanted to argue, she was growing even angrier.

"I *had* a legitimate question, Tatiana! I *am* a smart person!" Spit flew from my mouth, and I wiped it with the back of my hand.

"Tom. You do what I say, or I will divorce you. Understand, Tom?" Another breaking point in the marriage, except this time immediately evident. She was very calm, which scared me. When she went wild, at least I knew she was being irrational. "I prohibit you from ever calling Professor Bernstein again at home. Ever. Understand?" She started back down the stairs, accepting no further argument. Once she was out of earshot and I could no longer yell at her, her words sank in far more deeply than they would have had she stayed.

CHAPTER 44

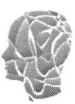

Smiley Faces

Tatiana meant well; she was trying to minimize the harm I was doing to my reputation. She knew firsthand the importance of a good relationship with one's graduate school mentors and wanted to help me preserve mine. I thought about what she had said.

Of course she was right, but I didn't want to admit it. Those days I felt I was always being told I was wrong. I didn't even know the full extent of what I didn't know. It was always surprising me. I was used to having an opinion that counted. Being regarded as unenlightened was difficult to get used to. Half the time I lost my temper because I felt insulted; just as often, I simply lost my cool.

Later during that fall of 1993, my psychiatric problems were under tenuous control with high doses of lithium and Serentil, but the toll on me in terms of energy—and, if I had recently taken my pills, mental dullness—was steep. I often went unshaven.

I could still type, though. I began to look in the newspaper for data entry jobs and soon found one at an insurance company, an hour's commute by bus, in a suburban office complex. My main difficulty was observing proper deference to my employer. At first, there was no problem; in fact, I won a promotion to headquarters downtown for making a backup of the data I was entering.

After I was transferred to the city office, though, I had to do routine semi-skilled work. At least I could take pleasure in a tree-lined two-mile walk through Brandywine Park before sitting in a cubicle for four hours each day, entering totals from insurance claims into a computer. I was overeducated.

Previously, working hard had meant I would be done sooner. Here, the more I applied myself, the more meaningless work I was given. It seemed as if I were rolling a rock uphill, only to have it roll back down. The job brought me face to face with the fact that I had no goals for my life, and I could not avoid the issue any longer. At least in school, I'd had the illusion of being productive because I was learning.

There was no chance for individual expression in the office besides the cubicle walls. Some of the female employees had decorated theirs with children's photos or crayon drawings. My immediate neighbor explained to me how he posted a little smiling doodle on a scrap of yellow sticky paper for every hundred reports he tallied successfully, and a frowning doodle for every report that came back with an error. The lower part of his cubicle walls was a chaos of happy doodles. He furtively explained to me that he was working on our boss's likeness in his unhappy doodles, which he had defiantly pinned facing her office at the top of his cubicle.

I felt as if I had been deprived of air. The creative student in me thought to try to rise above the situation and hope to be recognized. I began to work harder, remembering from school that time goes faster when one is lost in work. Break times made the rest of the hours tolerable. Then I could sit outside in a sunny courtyard and rejuvenate myself for another effort. Sometimes I would even find time for a brief walk.

As the cold weather came on, breaks were not as appealing. I was a strange clerk, willing to do some unskilled work but obsessed with how to get my boss to assign me different responsibilities. I convinced myself that if she and I did not see eye to eye, we could work something out.

I surreptitiously brought in Weber, the subject of my call to the professor, to read between spurts of activity. These pages were my connection to my former life. One day in the late fall I put in an extra-hard fifty minutes and, to test the waters, began to read some Xeroxed pages of my book. I strained at the effort through double vision. My neighbor saw what I was doing and whispered a sharp warning, but my actions had not escaped the attention of our boss, whose office faced our cubicles. She called me in.

"It looks like you need some more work, Tom," she began, unsmiling.

"As a matter of fact, ma'am, I've been thinking I've been working pretty hard recently," I started, but she was not interested in talking. I was told to clean out my desk the next day.

CHAPTER 45

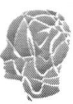

Think Fast

My neighbor posted an unhappy face with a pin through it for me. I confess that I was not entirely disappointed to be relieved of my duties, figuring that I now would have all the more time to spend on recovery.

At the same time, I began to volunteer at the mayor's office in Wilmington. An African-American professor from the University of Delaware, the mayor had recently won election, and I thought my recovery might benefit from working for him. A journalist friend had arranged an interview for me with the mayor's press secretary. My résumé reflected nothing of my injury and looked very impressive with my recent all-but-dissertation degree. I was soon offered a desk for weekly volunteer work.

Being at the mayor's office in the afternoons was the only high point of my day. Incidental projects would occasionally fall my way, chores I handled with pleasure. Once when a speech needed to be written on the spot and no one on staff was available for the job, I set about producing a first draft and came up with something reasonable in an unexpectedly short time. Soon it became known in the office that I had talent worth exploiting.

As my self-confidence grew that fall, I began to apply elsewhere for forty-hour-week jobs. Luckily, I was still able to drive. One firm offered me a research position that fit my background particularly well. I was to regularly travel to the Library of Congress in Washington, DC, and report back from my missions with summaries on what I had found. I was excited by the prospect of getting paid to do what I already did best.

My predecessor in the job had never finished his dissertation at Harvard. My own unfinished degree seemed to fit right in. "Are you sure you aren't interested in an academic career?" my interviewer asked.

"I've decided to be more practical," I said, faking certainty. I just wanted a regular paycheck for something I liked to do and said what came to mind. For the first time since my accident, I felt as if I was being treated as an equal among people interested in discussing ideas for their own sake. I felt empowered.

The writing test was an afterthought to my interviewers, and to me as well. It was simple: an encyclopedia, a few charts, a Xeroxed biographical blurb, and ten minutes to turn all of this information into a complete paragraph about a historical figure and his importance. I got stuck on the encyclopedia article. I began to read it, lost track of the flow after the first few sentences, then went back to the beginning. I read it again and forced myself to the end, losing concentration at approximately the same spot. I picked up pieces of scattered data as I floated my eye over the page and finished with a porridge of information in my head.

Why was I reading this article, anyway? What information was I looking for? I shoved the encyclopedia aside and tried to concentrate on the biographical blurb, hoping to find some clues there.

I looked furtively at my watch. Five minutes had passed. Half of my time was over, and I was still not following a lead. The looming certainty of my failure suddenly struck me and I began to panic. Beads of sweat formed in my armpits and rolled down my body, leaving thin tracks of coolness. I knew I had to start writing, or I would have nothing to show the committee. But writing only follows after material has been absorbed, and I had not taken in anything. Instead, I had just pushed my eyes over the page.

As I sat down at the black electric typewriter in the closed storage room and rolled a blank page into the carriage, I knew I couldn't produce anything. I had not digested the material—I hadn't even swallowed it. But I was too proud to show the committee a blank page. I began to type, copying words from the encyclopedia. I found the point of the first sentence of the article. Then I combined it in a sentence with the article's second sentence. Period. Then I looked at the biographical sketch. I summarized its first sentence. Period.

I looked at my watch. No time left. Again I was too proud to stay in the room longer than the time allotted. I rolled my feeble effort out of the typewriter and left the storage room to find the woman who had called me to the interview.

CHAPTER 46

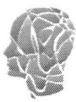

Rain

"I don't know what happened," I began, showing her my two sentences. "I just got stuck." Writer's block. A good excuse.

She tried to empathize. "Maybe some black coffee? Another ten minutes?" She seemed to have liked me in the interview and wanted to help with this formality.

But only I knew the full extent of my inability. No amount of time would help me in my condition, and coffee would only upset me further. "No, I only drink decaf," I said, obviously confused. I grabbed my umbrella. "I had a brain injury a while ago. Car accident," I said, falling back on the truth, the easiest path for those who can't think fast.

Her face registered shock. Suddenly she turned from a buddy-buddy intellectual to a professional interviewer. "Oh, well, thank you very much. We'll be in touch."

"Yeah, right," I thought. "In touch. I'll be awaiting the rejection letter in the mail, if you even bother to send one."

I walked from her office through a light rain to my car across the street, too distracted to open my umbrella. Fumbling angrily with the keys, I got in, slammed the door, and cried out at full volume. I screamed and cursed repeatedly, hitting my steering wheel at each word. I had come face to face with my disability. The rehabilitation therapists had warned me that this would happen. Was my life now to be full of moments like this? Was I to discover other surprise gaps in my functioning? I thought my recovery had been going so well.

I arrived home not wanting to face my father or Tatiana. But they were eager to hear news of my first real job interview. "How did it go, Tom?"

I shook my head in disbelief. In college I had written for major city newspapers. I was the author of an amendment to Haverford's student constitution. My old identity, though, no longer served me. "Something . . . I don't know . . . the writing test . . . went wrong . . . I don't get it . . . I couldn't do it . . . I don't get it."

They were stunned. Evidently they, too, thought I had been mainstreaming myself more successfully than I had. "What do you mean, Tom?"

My temper flared at their probing. I directed my pain toward Tatiana, the easiest target. "I don't know what I f*cking mean, Tatiana. I failed it, that's all!" I ran upstairs to my bed and threw myself face down. The silence of the room didn't help.

When I finally made my way downstairs, Tatiana sulked out of the room. My father gently reprimanded me for yelling at her. They had been talking. Neither of them was used to the outbursts of anger that I felt so free to aim at them. Whereas my father felt a certain paternal obligation to put up with me, Tatiana did not, and let him know she would not stand for abuse. New to the role of marital counselor, my father had tried to comfort her by saying that things would improve with time and therapy.

Disabled or not, with a temper like mine, I was unprepared for a job. The damage I was doing to my marriage didn't register with me, either. I went into the other room, flopped on the couch, and turned on the TV. I was too self-absorbed to apologize.

CHAPTER 47

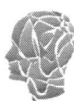

Pills From Tibet

Volunteering at the mayor's office once a week was good for my morale, but my real purpose in life was alternative medicine. I had heard of the Lotus Center near Newark, Delaware, and considered it worth looking into. It was a local outlet for many New Age services and products, run by a well-intentioned young man who had written a thesis at the local university about Eastern medicine and ever since had been convinced of its healing value. He had married a Chinese doctor, in the process finding a partner to make his products available by prescription.

The proprietor of the Lotus Center sat in on his wife's treatment sessions, like a medical student at a hospital, except he didn't ask the patient's permission first. I had taken a dislike to him, but his center was the only place I could see his wife.

On one of my visits that spring, the proprietor blocked the doorway of his wife's office as I was about to leave. In his hand was a vial, supposedly a great cure for emotional instability and head injury. Only fifteen dollars. "Well," I thought, "the worst that can happen is that it won't work."

At home I began to take regular doses of the remedy. It came dissolved in grain alcohol, the equivalent of a glass of wine for each dropperful. I should have learned in Moscow that insanity would be close on the heels of alcohol in any form, but I was too eager to cure myself and too stubborn to consider the possibility of error.

At home, after two days of the medicine three times a day, I was no longer sleeping and was beginning to talk of my return to graduate school, much to everyone's chagrin. I wanted to rent an apartment in New York with my savings. I had my thesis outlined, I thought, into chapters scattered around my disorganized desk upstairs. I simply was having trouble finding them.

My father kept remarkably calm as I told him of my plans. I felt free to express them to him, though, because he, unlike Tatiana, never lost his cool upon hearing them. He was steady enough that he was even volunteering at a crisis hotline. I had stopped mentioning my thesis to Tatiana. Any reference to it drove her berserk.

My father was seated at the kitchen table reading the newspaper as I elaborated. "Why don't you sit down, Thomas?"

"No, I like standing," I said. Hypomania, the excited condition preceding a manic episode, makes relaxation difficult. Considering the amount of sleep I had gotten during the seventy-two hours immediately prior, I should have crashed head forward onto the table.

Suddenly my eye fell on the medicine vial and my mind struck a spark. I grabbed the bottle and looked at its ingredients. "Holy cow, Dad! I'm losing it!" I gulped. "Dad, I need to see a doctor."

With tremendous effort, I forced myself to sit down. I learned afterward that most manic-depressive patients are not as self-aware as I am. Many of them even enjoy the rush of being hypomanic. I guess I'm lucky that I am scared of the psychosis that I know hypomania leads to. It almost killed me in Moscow.

Filled with dread, I bounced back out of the chair and called Dr. Spalding's office. Fortunately, it was a weekday and his secretary answered. "Linda, this is Tom Hartmann and I've just gone manic again, no kidding. What should I do? Could you have the doctor call me?"

To his credit, he called back within the half hour, and I jumped for the phone. I had been pacing along a path I had defined through the rooms downstairs, but once I picked up the receiver, the phone's cord limited me to shuffling up and down a short stretch of hall. I grabbed a loose pen and a sheet off a pile of scrap paper to write down his recommendation for a dramatic dosage increase. I wasn't second-guessing my doctor anymore, now that I was so clearly losing my sanity. To everyone's relief we managed to nip the crisis in the bud—early enough, in fact, that I didn't have to remain at that huge antipsychotic dose for more than a couple of weeks.

Close to five years later, after many panicked middle-of-the-night phone calls to doctors over sleeplessness, I finally learned to spot a disconnect with reality in its very early stages. I found that the only way to stop a psychotic attack before it took over was to be alert and ready to lose everything—daily routine, sleep cycle, plans, hopes for the foreseeable future—in order to maintain my sanity. More than likely, I would end up having to medicate myself into oblivion.

Being duped once at the Lotus Center did not stop me from seeing the Chinese doctor again. After all, I had committed myself to finding alternative cures for head injury—bipolarity, too—if there were any. I was convinced that I had to experiment, with myself as the guinea pig.

I was a little sedated during the next few Lotus Center visits but did not have the presence of mind to ask for a refund for the "miracle cure" that had almost derailed me. Both proprietor and doctor could not have helped noticing the drop in my quality of life that followed on the heels of their remedy. I suspect they appreciated my loyalty as a client and, in the end, my not hammering in their mistake probably worked to my advantage. I think they looked for a way to make it up to me, and the next time, we struck gold.

Not too long thereafter, I managed to see the doctor alone in her office. "Doctor Xing," I said, "I have trouble coming up with new ideas. Trouble reading, too. I've made great improvement since last year, but there's still something missing. I don't think the astragalus works anymore."

"You're right," she said. "Astragalus is only good for the first phase of recovery. But"—here she smiled—"while I was in China on my last visit, I met a Tibetan. He gave me some pills they use to treat people who have fallen off horses. Maybe they will work. I'll give them to you at no cost, because he gave them to me for free."

A horse accident did not seem like a far cry from a car accident to me. Evidently, the doctor thought the same. The big blue pills were packaged in silk envelopes, placed like six eggs in a small cardboard carton. Instructions were written in Tibetan and English on rice paper. I looked at the list of seventy ingredients, one of which was pearl. The directions were to dissolve in hot water and drink one pill a day. And to have no sex, no surprises, and not much exercise for a week.

My gut feeling was that these pills were safe to take. Tibet is so remote and has such a harsh climate that there is very little room for error in their arts. I tried my best to follow the instructions.

CHAPTER 48

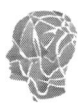

M&M's at the Orchestra

A week later, I had already forgotten that I had taken the Tibetan pills. I was sitting with Tatiana and her Russian friends at the kitchen table. It was something I had always loved to do. We had spent endless hours this way together in Bryn Mawr and New York. Russia, too. Just listening to conversation made me feel more intelligent than I was these days. For months, I had barely been able to follow the thread of their discussion, let alone contribute.

The topic was politics: Russian president Yeltsin had recently ordered his military to fire at Moscow's parliament building.

"Yes, but you know," I interjected, "democracy can only be achieved by democratic means. It's an important principle in political science." The women stopped their discussion to look at me. I hadn't spoken much for most of the past year, yet I had just said something interesting at an appropriate point. Tatiana looked at me for a few seconds in mute astonishment, and then turned back to her friends, confused.

One of them said, "He's right, you know. He's absolutely right. It was a terrible blow to Russian democracy, what Yeltsin did." This was the first compliment I had gotten on my intelligence since the accident, and it certainly meant more to me now than it would have in the past. I counted the months in my head: February 1993 to November 1993—almost a year.

I gave the Tibetan medicine credit. If it had worked for clumsy horsemen north of India for hundreds of years, why not for me? I returned to the Lotus Center the next day for more.

"Sorry, Tom, it was just an accident that I met this guy. Next time I go to China I'll see if I can find him."

My heart fell as I looked away. I could imagine myself searching a beach for one particular grain of sand. So my chances for a repeat of the Tibetan pills' success were less than one in a million. On the way home, though, my disappointment gradually turned to gratitude for this next little push toward recovery. "Synchronicity!" I smiled to myself, thinking of a favorite word. "I was in her office on the right day. And besides, every little bit more will build on what I have now."

This time I did not try to return to the rehab center to tell them that a cure existed for head injury. I remembered my resolution to quit wasting time trying to open other people's minds and shifted my focus to getting completely well, or at least recovered enough that my impressive gains would substantiate my claims of success.

I was still having trouble finding things to do with myself besides going to my volunteer job, seeing Dr. Spalding regularly, eating, sleeping, and taking my medicine. When my father saw me moping around the house, he was fast to point out that there were many small projects that needed to be done, but I wouldn't apply myself to them. Not only was I not handy, but for some reason I could no longer take much initiative.

Later, a different doctor would explain to me that in the brain, the thought of doing something—say, going downstairs to get a hammer—happens in one place, while the impetus to execute the intention—that is, actually stopping the present activity, walking over to the steps, going down them, and finding the hammer—comes out of a different location. He pointed out that my head injury had affected the location of that latter "executive function." In fact, it was no surprise that I spent hours lying on the couch talking about what I was going to do, but never even getting up.

Early the next year, in 1994, my father took me to hear the Philadelphia Orchestra. The program was an especially good one, and I was pleased to be doing something festive with my evening instead of staring at my wallpapered ceiling. As it turned out, my father enjoyed the music while I stared at the ceiling of the Academy of Music. I couldn't wait for intermission, and I couldn't stop thinking about what I would buy at the concession stand. All through the first, second, and final movements of the performance, my thoughts revolved around whether or not they would be selling peanut M&M's. Would they sell the extra-large package or just regular?

I moved uncomfortably in my seat, impatient for intermission, not even interested enough to keep track of the most basic contours of the beautiful sounds around me. I clapped when the others did, wondering each time whether it was appropriate now to get up and leave. I knew enough not to make a point of my utter inability to appreciate the music, or to even mention it to my father. In spite of the small strides that I had made, my boredom that evening made me aware that I still had much more recovering to do.

CHAPTER 49

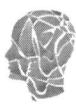

Shamanic Healing

As I became able to think more clearly, the emptiness of my life became more palpable. Maybe my father had mentioned my need for therapy to Dr. Spalding, or maybe in his office I let slip a nasty comment about my mother, but soon the doctor referred me to his associate psychologist for counseling. He felt that my weekly fifteen-minute medication checkups were not enough to deal with all aspects of my case.

The associate helped me realize that I had not cried much in the past fifteen years, and raised the question of whether my manic depression was part of a larger problem. Before my accident, I had been able to overcome most of life's obstacles with charm and wit. What would I do if I had to actually grow up and learn how to face the world without these tricks?

The first practical idea I got out of his therapy was to visit a men's group, a short-lived experiment in small-group intimacy, run by the same journalist friend who had gotten me the job interview at the mayor's office. I was lonely and drawn to its openness. Soon after, I quit therapy with the psychologist. Then a member of the men's group suggested that his acquaintance, a shaman, might be able to help me.

When we met and I found out that she did not ask for payment, I allowed myself to be convinced that she could do no wrong. I was ready for anything, certainly for this chance at recovery.

The shaman did have a magical presence about her. She lived in a row house in the city but did not lock her doors. The guy from the men's group told me that her husband was an Inuit Eskimo. "Inuit" caught my attention in the same way "Tibetan" had: thousands of years in harsh conditions probably made for no-nonsense medical practices.

Upon my first visit to her home, I was impressed by large, exuberant paintings in primary colors: her own artwork, I later found out. She was wearing a white jumpsuit, and her energetic eyes were set off by dark, flowing hair. She took me to her consultation room upstairs and exclaimed, "What a beautiful aura! Bright blue."

As I lay on her examination table, she placed her hands on both sides of my head and let her fingers rest on my scalp. Five minutes into the session, her breathing became more intense, and her fingers moved across the surface of my head as though she were trying to dig something out. About ten minutes later, she removed her hands and walked to a window, bent over, and held her ankles.

"What were you doing?" I asked, sitting up.

She pulled up a chair and began drawing a picture. "This is what your brain looked like to me," she said. She drew two adjacent hemispheres with a dent in the front of one of them. Without being told, she had precisely identified my injury: left frontal lobe damage. Ready to be persuaded, I was convinced she had some sort of special powers.

"I want to see you every month, and I recommend that you continue with your acupuncture." I did end up seeing her several times thereafter. Once she worked on healing a wound in my abdomen, left over from exploratory surgery immediately after the accident.

She also offered to do a "soul retrieval," gathering the pieces of my psyche lost over a lifetime of various traumas. The idea that my soul was in pieces made sense to me. Fragments could have split off during family upheavals, or because of school, to say nothing of bipolarity, brain injury, isolation chambers, or marital difficulties. I quickly agreed that a soul retrieval might do me some good. "It is intensely emotional work. There is some risk it could destabilize you," she told me.

At the next session I told her about my dream from the night before: a grizzly bear was chasing me down a mountain, and the only way I could hope to save myself was by turning around and wildly waving my arms to scare it off. She interpreted my willingness to confront death unarmed and confident as a sign that I wanted to undergo the retrieval. Many years later, I wrote her a thank-you letter for her decision. While it proved to be a journey through hell, I emerged a better person.

I entertained the thought that she might be able to cure my manic depression in one day. After all, shock therapy sometimes has instant success. Why not something more holistic? At her suggestion, I taped the session on a portable recorder so I would not forget what had happened. Lying on the floor next to me, she listened to Native American drumming and closed her eyes, letting rhythms and visualizations alter her mental state. Next to her, I looked at the ceiling, feeling nothing. After about ten minutes, she opened her eyes and slowly sat up across from me. "Let me tell you what happened," she said.

CHAPTER 50

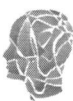

Descent Into Madness

On her journey through my dream world, she had first met a well-dressed, proud young man, who agreed to come with her as long as she acknowledged that he was confident and handsome. After she assured him that indeed both words described him, they went on together and eventually entered the emergency room of a hospital, where another young man was lying in a coma. "This is the man we must help," she said to her companion.

Then, in a nearby closet, she found a boy with an expressionless face who could not be persuaded to come with her. "I have no heart," he said. "I keep it locked away, so people can't hurt me." When she asked the boy to show her where he kept his heart, he took her by the hand and led her through a desert. There he dug up a locked box. She persuaded the boy to come back to the emergency room with the box. Then she woke up.

The shaman removed her headphones and carefully recounted the story, evidently trying to remember it properly as I remained silent. Unexpectedly, each of the separate individuals spoke to a certain part of me.

Now that I have been through long-term psychotherapy, I can see that the soul retrieval suddenly presented material that in session I would have uncovered only gradually. The single visit was remarkable for the scope of what it showed me. I thanked her, even though her exploration had put me into overload.

I felt pity for the boy in her story, and discomfort with the similarities between myself and the well-dressed young man. "What can I do to help that boy?" I asked her, feeling self-conscious at the extent to which my innermost self had been exposed to her intuitive eye. I felt that I had been denying a deficit in my life until she so deftly uncovered it in her story. Asking how to help the boy was a metaphor for asking how I could help myself.

"Be nice to him," she said. "Remember him in your life." She smiled. What more could she say? She had done her work.

Energized by the news, I came back home and played the recording of the session for Tatiana, who was unimpressed, especially when I took to playing it repeatedly. She had not taken a liking to the shaman. On my recommendation, she had gone for a soul retrieval herself and had been put off by some of what she had been told.

I impulsively made a trip to Ingeborg's and told her what had happened. She and I had been estranged before the accident, but during my recent time at home we had built up a tenuous bond. When I told her about my need to get in touch with my younger self, she was more than happy to dig out old photographs. She was looking for a way to get rid of them anyway. In these pictures, I looked happy, confident, and playful.

I looked at myself as a child and suddenly began to cry for the first time in recent memory, my whole body shaking, tears dripping onto the carefully mounted photos. The image of the boy locking his heart away, so vulnerable, seemed tragic and moving. Then to have the insult of disability added to the injury of abandonment . . . I felt sorry for myself for the first time since the accident.

I left my mother's with traces of tears on my face. I did not wipe them away, wanting to keep them as long as possible as testaments to my recent encounter with my emotions.

That night I had a lot of trouble sleeping. The red glare of my digital clock reminded me of the passage of about two hours as I tossed fitfully on the bed. Eventually I sprang up, squatted by my files, and obsessively arranged notes according to what I might need for my graduate research. My rummaging woke my father. Tatiana was away at Bryn Mawr. At five o'clock he opened the door to my attic apartment and asked in a tired voice if I was okay. "Sure," I answered breezily. "Just getting my papers in order." He was too tired to investigate the mystery further and went back to bed.

My energy seemed boundless. Evidently hypomania was once again underway. To my father's delight, my appetite was infinite. I ate three bowls of oatmeal with raisins at breakfast before returning to my room to clean up. It was normally a mess. I had spent the dark morning hours organizing and continued the huge job after my meal. This time I stayed away from Tatiana's things, remembering the book episode. I took special care in placing the photographs of myself as a child prominently on the desk. Around eleven o'clock, I began on the bathroom.

I could not stop moving or thinking. My activities were becoming more and more disjointed. In the middle of the bathroom cleaning, I suddenly felt no desire to continue. I paced the room and reflected. Suddenly it dawned on me that my fervent activity was reminiscent of some scary episodes not too long past. "Holy cow," I thought, just as I had before, "I'm becoming manic! I was fine yesterday, but now I've lost it." How could my sanity disappear so fast?

Adrenaline flooded my system. I ran downstairs to my father. Looking at him with wild eyes, I said in a shaky voice, "Dad, I think I'm going crazy again." He was the picture of calmness. "Okay, Thomas, I'll make an appointment with Doctor Spalding." We didn't yet know that, when a manic attack is beginning, every minute counts.

By this time Tatiana had arrived home. When I told her what was happening to me, she grew very serious. She looked me in the eye and said, "This is it, Tom. The last time. After this, I'm leaving you."

PART V

ON MY OWN

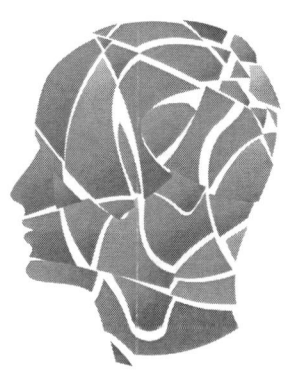

CHAPTER 51

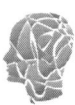

The Cuckoo's Nest Again

". . . At the sound of the tone, please leave a detailed message. Don't forget to mention the time you called, and please spell your last name . . ." The doctor could not be reached by telephone. It was a Friday, after all. "If this is an emergency requiring immediate attention, dial nine-one-one." I was already hanging up by the time that potentially lifesaving part of the message came on. Too bad.

My mother had tried to tell me once that there were two kinds of psychiatrists in Wilmington—the twenty-four-hour type, who is devoted to her patients, and the nine-to-five psychiatrist with a nice bedside manner, who would never inconvenience himself to be at the bedside. She was implying that I had employed the latter. Unfortunately our estrangement had kept me from listening to much of anything she had to offer, not that I could pick up on subtleties anyway.

It was February 1995. I was not confident enough to medicate myself, a very important skill in such a crisis, and by Monday my pills no longer helped. I got no sleep that weekend. By the time I saw the doctor in his office, I merely stared out his window, unblinking. "My mind"—I searched for words—"is like a desert . . ." He prescribed increased doses of all my medications, as he had the previous spring, but this time it was too late. Those pills should have been taken at the first signs of illness.

In the future, all of my psychiatrists would be surprised at how fast my sanity could slip away.

By Wednesday morning, my reality was unrecognizably fragmented, just like in Moscow. I was naked, chewing on a leather slipper, barking at my father and wife, and emptying all my medications onto the kitchen floor. Tatiana, not knowing what else to do, phoned Ingeborg and hoped for the best.

"Oh, that's her at the door!" called Tatiana, "Thank God!" My mother had agreed to come help get me to the hospital on the condition that my father would not be present. He took the occasion to handle some business and was not in the house.

I was in the living room, agitated, unable to contain what seemed like boundless energy. Tatiana, however, was already greeting Ingeborg out front.

"I've done my homework," said my mom in her can-do style. "The hospital is expecting him. We'll drive over, the three of us. And if there's a problem," I heard her add stiffly, "we'll call the police." She glanced into the living room from the entry hall. "Tom, my car's parked out front. Put on some clothes and let's go."

It was lucky that I hadn't knocked over any furniture, let alone my father's artwork, while jumping around the room, doing modified calisthenics. I was reciting some Russian children's poetry I remembered from college and wore a pleased expression.

"Tom, they're waiting for us. You need to get your things." Tatiana had warned Ingeborg she was most likely to be successful if she dealt with me matter-of-factly and respectfully.

Surprisingly, maternal authority still had some effect. After I kept them waiting for a few moments, something in me clicked. "Okay! No problem!" I pulled on the sweatshirt and pants that were lying on the bench and stopped running in place. "Are my shoes out there on the shoe rack?" We always left them at the door in my father's home; I'm not sure if that was due to oriental influence or if he just didn't want dirt on the floor. Tatiana and Ingeborg waited in silence while I laced up, not bothering to suggest that I put on socks.

Wilmington Hospital was only about ten minutes from my dad's home. Tatiana and I sat in the back of my mom's white Pontiac, Tatiana holding my hand supportively as I fidgeted.

We did not go to the emergency room; regular Admissions in the main lobby would do. As my mother had promised, they were expecting me. The woman at the desk called the floor, and as we finished Xeroxing insurance cards, someone came up from the psychiatric ward to usher me back. I was completely absorbed in myself, concerned only with the chaos in my mind. I didn't say goodbye and couldn't really understand the import of Tatiana's last words to me: "I'm going back to Moscow after this."

* * *

As I passed through the ward's doors, some recollection of my previous isolation must have kicked in because I began to count to ten in three languages at the top of my voice. The staff decided to assign their only bilingual psychiatrist, a German, to my case. Then I was hurried off to isolation.

Raving lunatics are often brought onto psych wards. Invariably they are carted off to isolation, just as I was. However, at this new hospital, I was locked in a room behind an antechamber with a toilet, which provided a buffer zone, thus allowing the floor to remain peaceful in spite of my shouting and making for a quieter atmosphere than I had experienced to date.

It was a relief to be hospitalized where the staff were conscious of how to handle patients humanely. I was not thinking in words at that point, but in many ways my awareness was heightened. Although I was hard to reason with due to insanity, I never had the sense of being threatened or condescended to. That was a pleasant change from previous hospitalizations.

I am just as glad that I have few memories of this most recent time in isolation, save a hazy recollection of being allowed to use the toilet with orderlies in the room. It's disablingly difficult to go to the bathroom in public. They were evidently afraid that I might harm myself. As far-fetched as it seemed, the doctor had asked my father to ransack my possessions for any sign of suicidal tendencies, and, after combing my files and journals, some dating back more than ten years, Dad had returned with what might have been a suggestion to that effect. At the time, I had no idea I owed all this excessive oversight to some supposedly private scribbling.

CHAPTER 52

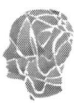

"I Am the Idiot"

The heightened security during toilet time may actually have saved my life. Habitually an upbeat and confident guy, I began to wonder during my time in isolation if all life held for me, ultimately, was one straitjacket after another. Though there had been high points, it seemed to me that my two previous years were headed nowhere, and I knew I was wearing down my dad and Tatiana.

Dr. Bergman, the German psychiatrist, visited me daily to check out my progress and look for clues as to how to handle my case. By the ninth day in the isolation chamber, I just wanted out. I remember the sensation of floating aimlessly in a vast and cold space with no frame of reference, as if I were a far-off planet that had just lost touch with the sun's gravitational force. I no longer felt the pull of my family, of a daily routine, or of my wife.

Not finding any way of grounding my mind but no longer physically tied down, I scanned the room for some way to get out. There were no windows, so I couldn't jump or climb out, and Dr. Bergman was in the doorway talking to someone with his back to me, effectively blocking the exit.

As I looked at him, the toilet in the antechamber came into focus and presented itself to me as a body of water I could lose myself in. Clumsily I got off the stretcher and shambled over to it. When I was a few feet away, I lunged for the bowl, plunging in my face. Before I could gag, I felt pain at the back of my head. Hey, that hurt!

"I got him, Dr. Bergman! He's alive for sure," someone called out triumphantly. What was going on? Water poured out of my nose as I reached up to claw at the orderly's hand, which still held a handful of my hair.

Dr. Bergman must have appreciated the quick reflexes that had saved his patient, but he was fast to give his assistant a dressing down for handling me roughly. "Always use as little force as possible. Watch," he said, using the opportunity to demonstrate how to handle me by bending down himself and gently taking me by the shoulders. I coughed up more water.

Eventually, after several days, the doctor got my pills right and I came to. I later learned that he had made a special research trip to find out the best known combination of medicines for bipolarity and traumatic brain injury, something I very much appreciated, even though his findings took him to the same conclusion Dr. Schwein had reached: lithium and Serentil. So, out I came from isolation.

The new doctor visited me in my private room every working day. He had an office in the hospital and slept there when necessary. On account of my insanity during my stay to date, the patient he had encountered so far was not actually me, just a shadow of myself. By the time we really met I had impressed the staff as an exemplary patient, a far cry from the me who, only a week and a half earlier, had needed six orderlies to hold him down.

The first thing any psychotherapist wants to know is why the patient is there. The answer to that question lets the patient express himself and allows the doctor to get a feel for the person he will be working with as well as a basis for therapy. But how the doctor asks that first question tells the patient a lot about the doctor, and I liked Dr. Bergman from the beginning because of his friendly and unpretentious manner.

Unlike Dr. Schwein's cold "So, tell me your case history," or even Dr. Spalding's studied "What seems to be the problem?" or his negatively phrased "What do you think is wrong with you?" Dr. Bergman's warm "Tell me about yourself" awakened a willing and hopeful response.

I told him the first thing that crossed my mind, something that seemed to say a lot about me.

Making myself quite vulnerable, I told him that the closest parallel I could think of in literature to describe my personality was Prince Myshkin of Dostoevsky's book *The Idiot*. In the novel, a noble yet simple man is mistaken for a fool and ends the book in a mental hospital. The story had spoken to me directly when I read it the first time. "I'm the idiot," I confided to him, speaking with the intimate honesty of close friends who have let down their guard.

The surprising thing was not that I expressed myself with a literary analogy. This suited my normal personality. More astounding was that the doctor knew Dostoevsky's novel and knew the character. He had read it as part of the formal education he received in Germany. In addition to being a very capable psychiatrist, he was a cultured man, something experience had led me to believe was a rare combination in America.

"Yes, Tom, I understand. But Prince Myshkin dies in the end. We don't want you to die," he said with a smile. "Well, we'll continue our talk tomorrow. See you later." End of session one.

I smiled goodbye as he left my room. "Wow! What a change!" I thought, feeling as jubilant as anyone on Serentil could hope to feel. "Doctor Bergman seems to really like me. I think my stay here is going to go well."

My biggest concern as I came into full consciousness was that the life I had been putting together for myself over the past months was pretty surely in pieces after this most recent bout with psychosis. The routine of daily work at the mayor's office had been broken, and with it had gone my feeling of dignity and self-worth. I was no longer an aide to someone important, rather a mentally ill person soon to emerge from a locked ward. My identity in the world outside had been wiped away by the unexpected power of a shaman.

Then a package of fruit arrived from my "Friends at the Mayor's Office." My heart melted. How did they know that fruit was my favorite food? I finished it off in less than two days. The fact that they still thought of me at the workplace helped to reestablish my self-respect. One evening my boss even dropped by to see me. Visits connected me with the world outside the hospital and made me feel like a healthy man who had had an accident, not a sick man relapsed into a chronic condition. I became anxious to get out and make a new start.

This time, putting the pieces of my life back together after my stay in the mental hospital was easier than I had thought it would be, largely because I had a work routine to provide me with structure and moral support. I was accepted back at the office as though nothing had happened.

CHAPTER 53

Busted

Several months after my release, my father was again given a pair of tickets to hear the Philadelphia Orchestra, this time at their outdoor summer venue. I accepted his invitation, mostly for lack of anything better to do, and partly from a curiosity about whether I could sit through an entire performance without becoming restless the way I had at the Academy of Music the previous year. As it turned out, I found the concert delightful.

"Dad," I said while we were clapping, "this was a great program and what's more, I could really appreciate the music this time. Maybe you didn't realize it, but when we went to the Academy I was too brain damaged to even listen." Perhaps he had realized and just hadn't mentioned it. "I can tell I'm getting better," I added enthusiastically.

"Maybe, Tom, maybe," he said noncommittally.

"So," I thought, "he's not setting great store by anything exciting I have to say about myself." I didn't have the presence of mind to see my situation from his perspective: ever-optimistic Tom, delighted with every step he's taken along a thousand-mile journey. I had the vague sense that my previous proclamations had lost me credibility, but the only way I knew how to compensate was by showing more enthusiasm. At least he wasn't expressing active doubts to me.

* * *

"Tomsik, I hope you are okay. The pace of life at the *dacha* is almost dreamy, it is so slow. My father is always up at dawn, you remember, writing. We collect mushrooms in the afternoons . . ."

True to her word, Tatiana had decided to take the summer to recuperate in Moscow. It was 1995, the Internet had recently come into general use, and we remained loyal to each other with daily electronic messages. Through Tatiana I had met Anna, one of her Russian friends in Wilmington, and I was glad for a little social life. A circle of Russian émigrés had developed around Anna, and I fell in with them easily while Tatiana was away.

She returned in August of 1995, hardly recovered. She had not carried through on her threat to leave me when I went insane again; instead, she was forcing herself to operate under an unbearable strain. I don't even know if she came back by her own choice or in response to her father. His decree to be loyal to me evidently had enormous influence. Within a few weeks after her return, she had a nervous breakdown.

When the policewoman called, I was in my father's home. "This is the New Castle County Police. We have your wife," she said. "She does not want to speak to you, but this is the number she gave us."

"Let me talk with her, please," I said.

I heard Tatiana's sobbing voice. "Don't be angry at me, my dearest. My dearest Tom, please." She sobbed again.

"My dear, what happened?" I asked.

"I stole some clothes. I was very bad. They were worthless cheap clothes. I wanted them to catch me, Tom. I want to go to jail. I am bad, Tom. Don't come to get me, please. I want to suffer." She sobbed again.

"I'll be right there, dear. Don't go anywhere."

"Please don't come, Tom."

* * *

I pulled open the glass door of the one-story New Castle County Police headquarters.

"First master's degree I ever arrested," mumbled the police officer as I entered.

Tatiana was curled in a brown plastic chair, holding her knees. She wore a blue long-sleeved T-shirt and black-and-white-striped leggings. She looked like an American.

My father had driven me to the station but remained at the entrance, not wanting to get involved. "Not him," she whispered to me in Russian. She did not like her authoritative German father-in-law and she seemed scared now. He could be harsh at times without intending to be. Warmth and tolerance for disorder come naturally to most Russians, whereas Germans tend to be more distant and disciplined.

"What do we do now?" I asked Tatiana.

"I'm waiting for the judge. She's going to send me to jail. I know she will. Tom, I don't want to go to jail!" Tatiana threw her arms around me and cried. "Why did I steal those stupid clothes? I couldn't help it!" She started heaving again with sobs.

I waited with her, dumbstruck. To find such a sensitive, refined, tender soul in such raw surroundings was horrifying. What if she were sent to jail? I held her and waited.

When called, Tatiana insisted that I stay outside. She did not want the full ugliness of her condition made public with me present. I insisted on joining her, hoping that my sad and reverential husbandly expression might help the proceedings.

We entered the adjacent courtroom and waited. The room was dark and held about thirty seats facing a raised desk and leather chair. I was relieved to see an older woman in robes enter by a separate door. I hoped we could expect a lighter judgment from a woman who might be a mother than we could from a young man.

The judge looked down at Tatiana over her spectacles. "I understand that you stole two blouses, some socks, and some perfume at T. J. Maxx today. Why did you do that?" The judge tried to look unsympathetically at Tatiana, something I have always found hard to do. Even the judge was having difficulty, it seemed. It was clear that the case before her was something more than simple shoplifting.

"I wanted to go to jail," Tatiana whispered, looking at the floor.

"They would tear you apart in jail," answered the judge quickly. "You don't want to go to jail. I'm going to fine you for stealing, and I never want to see you here again. Do you understand? Or next time maybe I will send you to jail." She slammed her casebook closed and looked harshly over her glasses.

I think Tatiana was relieved, but I'm not sure. I took her under my arm and we walked out of the station together.

"Needs therapy," observed my father curtly as I climbed into the passenger side of his new Toyota Camry. I flashed him an astonished look. Tatiana lay in the back seat with her knees curled up around her chest.

Two days later we were in the courthouse once more. The judge peered over her glasses again, genuinely surprised. "I thought I said I never wanted to see you in here again," she said, looking down at Tatiana. She had just been arrested for shoplifting again, at the same store, by the same policewoman. This time she had stolen panties and toothpaste.

Tatiana looked at the floor. "I'm sorry. I won't do it again. I'm seeing a psychiatrist. He's given me pills." She was genuinely afraid of going to jail. She had been moved by an impulse to steal that she could not control.

"Let me see," said the judge. Tatiana took the bottle out of her purse and showed it to her. The judge looked at it and handed the bottle back. "If you do it again, I won't have any choice but to lock you up for thirty days."

"Will this be on my record forever?" Tatiana asked quietly.

"When you appeal to have it taken off your record, ask for me," said the judge compassionately. She was no longer trying to be intimidating. "Pay the fine at the window," she said, knocking her gavel against its wood. "Get well soon," she said as we left the courtroom.

I was still getting over the shock of the second phone call from the courthouse. "Don't say anything to me, Tom," Tatiana said in a steady voice. "It won't happen again. I'm going back to Russia."

We got into my small car and started to drive home. "I can't deal with America anymore. I think I'm stealing because I feel so empty, like I don't have anything to hold onto. Tom, it's like a black hole. Nothing could fill it. If I ever feel better I'll come back." She wasn't carrying out a threat to leave me—she was saving her sanity.

As we drove in silence, I turned her words over in my mind. It was as if a trapdoor had opened in the core of my being and I was in free fall. I wanted to argue, to complain, to persuade, but felt as if even the gentlest words might break her. "Do what you need to do," I whispered. "I'll be here for you." I was not sure that I was telling the truth. I knew too much about myself and loneliness.

She threw her arms around my neck and uncorked a stream of sobbing. "Tom, I did all I could. I tried my hardest. The only good that's come out of the past six years is your recovery. That's all I have to show for being here. Tom, my life is a failure." She fell back onto her seat and continued crying.

"Go back to Moscow, Tanya," I said calmly, stroking her arm. "I'll be here for you when you get back." I drove home, talking myself gently into a life of sacrifice and devotion as I ministered to her. I felt noble, little considering how often she had had the same conversation with herself on and off for the past year and a half since the accident—even the past four years, counting the onset of my insanity—and had chosen to minister to me. She pressed my hand and said, "Tom, you are my dearest. I have never loved anyone like I love you. Thank you." She wiped her tears away as we drove home through Wilmington's suburbs.

Soon after she left, my volunteer work at the mayor's office turned into a part-time job writing short letters to answer citizen complaints and doing research. Now I had to get up every morning, put on a tie, shave, and stay awake for several hours. This was no small challenge for someone who had been out of the hospital for just three months, but to some extent I could fall back on the fact that I was among my "Friends at the Mayor's Office." At least once a week I would call in to work and ask for another hour to get ready. Always desperately trying to make it in on time, I quickly became addicted to caffeine.

In December of 1995, Tatiana returned to the US for a month's visit. It was entirely too short. I had just gotten used to her presence when she had to leave again. But I had lost none of my resolve to maintain my end of our overseas romance. Pictures of her peeked at me over the loose papers on my desk. I talked of her proudly to my colleagues. Almost every day she sent a new e-mail and I tapped out a reply. In my mind there was no question that Tatiana and I could keep our marriage alive indefinitely.

CHAPTER 54

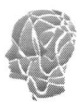

Farewell

By the spring of 1996, I was desperate for Tatiana's company. I also thought that a trip to Russia and time with her professor father would be good for my graduate ambitions. When I told Carter, my Haverford cycling friend, of my plans, he observed, "You're stepping back into the jaws that almost ate you." After all, he had been the one who arranged my father's ticket to Russia during the coup attempt.

Dr. Spalding was supportive, though. "Two weeks, eh? Well, just be careful about crossing so many time zones in one day. Take time to rest up." He pulled out his prescription pad. "You know not to push yourself. How many hours does the trip take?"

"Thirteen," I said. He stopped writing to shake his hand.

"Thirteen! Who-o-oa, writer's cramp." He finished the last prescription and handed them to me. "Don't wave all of these papers at once at the pharmacy," he joked, "or they really will think you are crazy.

"I'm giving you three copies for each script," he continued. "Carry one copy of each with you. The airline may ask you to show them. And pack so that you have a full set of pills in your suitcase, but in case it gets lost, keep another in your carry-on, and for good measure, do you have a fanny pack?" I nodded. "Keep an extra set there. You want to have enough in case you need to up your dosage. Foreign travel can get hairy."

"If anyone can relax, it's me," I assured him.

"So, take it easy and enjoy yourself. And if you have any trouble," he added, "tell my secretary to call me out of session. Don't worry, I'll be here." His confidence inspired mine.

I was lucky he actually was there when I did have to call.

* * *

That summer, in 1996, I visited Tatiana's family in Moscow, armed with all those pills and determined to keep my sanity.

Tatiana's mother and I were out buying fruit. I had been commenting on the availability of food these days, recalling citizens lined up for hours outside stores hoping something would be left on the shelves when it was their turn to shop. We had just breezed through the market and were already out on the sidewalk, each carrying a bag. The quality of life had improved noticeably in just a few years.

"The plums are great this season," I commented, slurping and spitting out the seed. Plums were Tatiana's favorite, but I snuck one from the bag. "Under the new system I guess they're able to import them so people can actually eat them." After a moment I added, "The first time Tatiana came to the US, she was amazed at the availability of produce, but when I get well and she comes home again, she'll probably take it all for granted."

"Yes," said Tatiana's mother, "if your marriage actually does work out, there are lots of things she likes about life in America. I do, too. You can see she'll always love fruit!" She was feeling chatty.

My head started spinning shortly after she began speaking. We kept walking, but my ears stopped off and I could barely hear her through a high-pitched ringing. I was stunned. She had said "if your marriage works out," not "when you get back together."

"If." It had not occurred to me that there was any possibility of our not working something out, even if it took a while. "If." How long had Tatiana's mother wondered whether we would ever get back together? Was it possible that she doubted it? Had Tatiana told her, but not me, that she, herself, doubted it? Surely Tatiana wasn't having real misgivings, but then again, her mother was her confidante . . . If I couldn't count on her mother to speak up in my favor, I was lost.

Looking back, I see that for Tatiana, there had been lots of times over the previous six years when her faith in our marriage had been shaken, starting with my trip to Germany shortly after our wedding and continuing through the car accident and the uncomfortable end of her most recent visit.

"If." Her mother's words pierced my heart. For the first time, it seemed plausible that our life together was doomed. By alluding to the possibility of failure, her mother had all but pulled out the cornerstone of everything Tatiana and I had created together, and it was starting to tumble down. I tried to put what now seemed like impending disaster out of my mind, but it kept surfacing, making me acutely aware of all of the dissatisfactions, large and small, Tatiana had ever voiced about me.

I knew that at this point Tatiana would want no part of my graduate "fantasies," as she now called them, but I was honestly hoping to consult with her father about the thesis I was still convinced I would soon be assembling, and hoped I could do so without making her worry that I was coming unhinged.

Sergei was fascinating, in part because original ideas sprang easily from his lips, ready to be explored. Sometimes he would spin them out in ways that delighted the minds of all who listened. Often he left it to others to follow up on his insights. I had been drawn in by a particular notion of his, that Stalin had kept his finger on the pulse of the Soviet empire through citizens' letters to him, and I thought just talking to Sergei about the idea would inspire me. He might even be able to point me toward some original documents. Maybe letters had been preserved somewhere.

In Moscow that summer, I sat at Sergei's kitchen table, the same table at which Tatiana and I had sat after my first "consultation" with him eight years before, the same table at which I had demanded holy water for cleansing when my mania had first bloomed five years before, the same table where her family had prepared food to bring to me in the mental hospital the summer of the coup, and the same table where the intelligentsia of Moscow had gathered for Bible study every Saturday during the years of the dictator Brezhnev.

Again I was warmed as Tatiana and I sat intimately with her parents, this time discussing her plans for work in Moscow. Tatiana wanted a real job after all those years of study, and Russia was a much better place for her to find one than America, where the best she could do was teach. Just listening to her interact with her brilliant stepfather delighted me, partly for old times' sake, but more because two sharp minds bantering over philology was my idea of fun. I felt like an admiring spectator at a ping-pong tournament. It made me forget how dulled my mind now was.

Implicit in Tatiana's job search was her expectation of staying in Moscow for the foreseeable future, but I didn't process that fact and only smiled at the high-level entertainment provided by the repartee.

Most of the lighthearted conversation actually centered on the subtleties of words, but before they were done, Sergei managed to convey how disappointed he was that she wasn't planning an academic career. I was proud to see her respectfully defend her aspirations in front of her father. Challenging his will, I knew, was difficult for anyone.

"So, you want to write about Stalin?" asked Sergei, turning his attention to me. "I'll think about it. Talk to me at the *dacha*. I'll give you a dissertation that should interest your people in the West." Russian academics like to believe that they are greater thinkers than their Western counterparts. At that, Sergei got up to go to his study, his wife rose to do the dishes, and Tatiana and I fell into conversation about what to do that evening.

Tatiana was in her element: her father had just confidently promised to change the career of yet another aspiring scholar at her kitchen table. She had seen it happen so many times that we even used to joke about her household being one of the centers of Russia's intellectual life. But even as we spoke, I wondered whether it could really be so easy for me to overcome what had already been years of brain injury. I had dreamed of the sort of *deus ex machina* that his words seemed to promise.

My exhilaration made me sleep poorly that night, but I told no one, hoping that a weekend of relaxation at the *dacha* would take the edge off my vigilant mind. The following night I loaded myself up with enough drugs to take care of most problems that could arise with my sleep, but I was already eating into my reserve stash.

Sergei, with a private bathhouse on his property, lived a life of relative luxury during his two months off from the university. In the city, Russians had to make do with the public baths. While in the country that summer, I slept alone out in the sauna's entryway. Tatiana was so traumatized by my history of middle-of-the-night ravings that she did not want me sleeping with her.

In the mornings, Sergei wrote, at a rate of seven pages per day. "Habit," he explained to me, an astounded novice who wrote a few paragraphs on a good morning. "Familiar material."

In the afternoons the family took walks in the adjacent forest, hunting for mushrooms. I understood this Russian national pastime poorly and did not try to compete with Tatiana and her parents. Requiring as relaxed a pace as possible, the Zen-like mushroom hunt trains the eye while whetting the appetite for the evening meal. I loved to join my in-laws and participate in the walk, if not the search.

After our walks, Sergei cooked lunch. His extensive knowledge of China included the cuisine, and he was a fabulous chef. He was a terrible sexist, though, who left all of the cleanup to his wife, and spent the late afternoons sunning himself and indulging in academic chat, sometimes dictating my dissertation questions to me. He was astoundingly familiar with the classic, if not the very latest, Western academic writings, and tried to help me understand how he had reconceived everything worth knowing about culture in his most recent book.

Once in the afternoon he showed me how to use his "lawn mower," the Russian version of a Weedwacker. It was a long-handled scythe, like the one carried by the Grim Reaper. "You must stand in one location and pivot, always keeping the blade parallel to the ground." He demonstrated, then let me try. I developed such a love for manual lawn mowing that at my next home I cut the grass using no power tools.

My official advisor in graduate school had been no help before my accident and was now hardly available to me, so I appreciated the firm direction that Sergei offered. His giving me a dissertation topic was a sign of paternal affection. We worked together in the sunny afternoons at the *dacha* until I thought I had the topic memorized.

In 1996, I couldn't concentrate very well and didn't think quickly enough to question complex ideas, but the didactic, charismatic, and somewhat self-centered professor enjoyed thinking. He overlooked my obvious deficits as a student and dictated his ideas into a tape recorder for me. Unfortunately, the accident had made my mind porous enough that even immediately after hearing his explanations, I couldn't conjure up essential concepts to serve as a framework for his words.

Looking back on my notes, I have difficulty reconstructing Sergei's logic, which, while it seemed faultless as he expressed it, was hard for me to capture on the page, and the recordings only make sporadic sense to me now.

I still regret losing the opportunity to nail his ideas down. As we discussed one exciting thing after another, my mind ran wild.

Working with him affected my sleep. My drugs no longer knocked me out for eight hours as I lay on the bench just inside the sauna. I slept or at least dozed perhaps half of that time, but lay starkly awake for the balance. I tried not to scare Tatiana but asked if we could return to Moscow soon so I could call Dr. Spalding.

Tatiana froze at my suggestion. "What's wrong?" she asked, her whole body tense.

"Nothing. I just want to prevent something from happening," I said.

"You're going crazy again, aren't you? Aren't you? Why didn't you tell us? We should never have come to the *dacha*. I knew it. Tom, I'm too weak." As she sobbed, I tried to cut in, to reassure her, but she was lost, visualizing certain doom. "This time there won't be the KGB chief's daughter at the mental hospital. This time it's Russian conditions. This time you're on your own. Oh my God!" She held her hands up to both sides of her head. "I tried my best. I tried my best," she said, with anguish in her voice. Dazed, she walked around in circles.

"Tatiana, I just want to return to Moscow to call Doctor Spalding as soon as possible. Nothing is going to happen today or tomorrow," I said calmly. Usually the lack of a phone made for a peaceful atmosphere at the *dacha*, but at that moment, its absence contributed to a low-grade panic. I assumed the role of her comforter in the midst of my own crisis.

Tatiana's mother was a steadying influence, my partner in an attempt to maintain levelheadedness in a deteriorating situation. I knew from prior experience that without help I would be insane in a matter of days. We all knew the possible consequences. We took the next train to Moscow.

Back in their apartment, I spoke on the phone with Linda, Dr. Spalding's secretary. It was 7 p.m. in Moscow, still before noon in America. "Linda, this is Tom. I'm calling from Moscow. Could you call Doctor Spalding out of session, please?"

"Moscow? It sounds like you're calling from just down the street!"

"Linda, please. It's a semi-emergency."

"Just a moment."

"Yes?" asked Dr. Spalding, carefully not saying my name in front of anyone in the room with him. "How're you doing?"

"Doctor Spalding, I'm not sleeping. What should I take?"

"Do you have trazodone?"

"Yes."

"Take trazodone, up to four hundred and fifty milligrams. Okay?"

"Okay. Thanks. Bye, Doctor Spalding."

"Bye, now. You sound great from here."

In a few days I was sleeping fine. Tatiana, though, could not sleep a wink. Her earlier traumas had been scratched open and lay raw. My two-week stay in Moscow had set her back immeasurably. When I left soon after, she was sad but grateful that I was going. Our marriage was in shreds.

CHAPTER 55

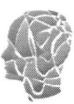

Stretched Too Far

Back home, despite the sunny weather, a suspicion that my life with Tatiana was beyond repair gave my days a bleak cast. We continued our loving e-mail correspondence and I did my best to keep my sanity. I maintained the increased medication Dr. Spalding had recommended and kept as structured a routine as possible, getting up to an alarm, shaving, working, taking walks, eating with my dad. I visited friends in the neighborhood, and after a while my life took on a nice pace.

Later that summer, I participated in a workshop for young Friends at a nearby Quaker retreat center. The atmosphere inspired intimacy among participants. Already an open person, I shared my secrets with all who cared to ask.

"She doesn't accept your illness? Your own wife?" asked a young woman as we strolled to the dining room.

"No, I don't either. When I am better, we'll be able to get back together again." This was the answer I had talked myself into, and it was what I told everyone. I did not know I was talking to another person who had bipolar disorder.

At my words, my companion suddenly swung in front of me and looked me in the eyes. It turned out that she had been in my position before.

"Tom, I know this is hard to accept, but you're never going to get better. Learn to live with it. And find someone who can accept you. You're twenty-nine. You've got a life to live." Her eyes pierced into mine. I could tell she was talking from painful experience.

She turned away and left me standing alone, unexpectedly jarred. I suddenly wanted to be held, to feel safe. I was stretching myself across the ocean via the Internet and semiannual visits. Get on with my life? My tie with Tatiana, already pulled too tightly, snapped apart like a rubber band.

The retreat lasted three more days. I was happy for the distraction. Although it had already been more than three years since my head injury, I was not yet able to maintain concentration for more than a few minutes, so the structured activities offered me welcome continuity. During meals and evening hours I still enjoyed conversation with the other participants.

The "Quaker girl," as I thought of her, didn't bring up manic depression or my failing marriage again, but she did shoot me significant glances, as if to remind me not to forget my situation.

After the retreat, I sent Tatiana an e-mail. "I cannot stand my loneliness," I wrote. "It's my fault that I'm so lonely, but I cannot exist in our marriage much longer unless you come home." I didn't even pause to ask myself if Wilmington was really her home. I knew that I was asking the impossible.

"Tom, my dear, I need years to recover," she wrote back. I pictured her face when she had asked if I was going crazy again, only a few weeks before. Would that panic ever dissipate or would it always be there, just below the surface? Maybe it would take years.

"Have an affair. I give you permission. Just don't catch anything."

The idea of having an affair was too alien. My problem was emotional, not physical. My loneliness was too deep for an uncommitted relationship.

I wrote back: "Tatiana, I can't go on like this. I am too needy. I want a divorce if you cannot come back." It was difficult to say who had suffered more in the last few years or whose life was more ruined. "Tanya, you have sacrificed everything for me. I am so weak and selfish."

Acceptance of personal suffering—almost the expectation of it—is part of the Russian character, but it was not part of mine. I felt guilty making a decision based on my own pain. She was ready to continue a postal marriage *ad infinitum* and was grieved that I wasn't. The drama was heart wrenching. It would never have occurred to either of us that our marriage had deteriorated into an unrealistic illusion and that it was better and healthier for both of us to let go. But she was in love with someone who no longer existed, and I didn't want to be left out in the cold.

She had come to a determination by the next night. "Tom, if you truly ask this of me, you can never come back again."

The strength behind her words gave me pause. It was hard to imagine that I could I ever find as deep a love as I had felt with her. I wanted to see if it was possible to find a new partner to sustain me now that she would very likely never return from Russia, but there was no way I could stand to find out in the context of an affair, whether or not she "gave me permission."

The power of my loneliness overcame my desire to be comforted every night by an e-mail or by the distant hope that Tatiana would someday find the strength to return to America. I never really considered moving to Russia. Crossing more than one time zone, I had learned, destabilized me badly enough that I needed to sedate myself beyond recognition.

Getting past loneliness became my life's primary goal, alongside healing my dual diagnosis of manic depression and brain injury. I had been lonely for as long as I could remember and had all along made a concerted effort to fulfill myself through the company of others. The loss of daily communion with Tatiana would, I knew, leave a gaping hole in my heart. It would be years before I learned to find sustenance from my own resources. Could I take a plunge alone into the unknown?

I wrote her that I wanted a divorce.

CHAPTER 56

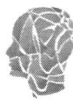

First Date

Tatiana and I would remain friends. My father was disappointed but not really surprised. He felt that Tatiana had left me in my time of need. I saw it differently: I had not been wholly appreciative of her during our brief marriage, and she had left only because she could not stay any longer. On the other hand, my mother saw it as a good solution. She, the militant feminist, was an advocate of divorce to solve all marital problems.

My tender nightly e-mail gone, I turned to the company of various other women I already knew.

I was happy to spend time with Tatiana's friend, Anna. I knew Anna wasn't interested in striking up a romance with me, but having a female friend who knew Tatiana made my loss less poignant. I knew that Anna missed Tatiana, too, and enjoyed talking about her. Besides, as a single mother, she could understand my disappointment at not having a mate. Soon I was a frequent visitor and even began to tutor her son in arithmetic.

Several times when I dropped by, I interrupted Anna while she was playing with her pet parakeet. She would nuzzle him and put him back on his perch, where he would warble affectionately. At least it sounded sweet to love-starved me. "I think I need a parakeet too," I told her once, "to keep from being alone so much of the time. What do you think? Or maybe a canary?" She burst out laughing. "What, a parrot?" I asked.

Still laughing, she told me to take a dinette chair. "Tom, birds may have soft feathers, but they have beaks and claws! You don't need a bird," she said. "You need a woman!"

She was right. With poorly concealed desperation, I began to look for a steady, local, female partner. First I turned to one of my neighbors, an attractive young professional. My calls were coolly ignored.

Then, another neighborhood acquaintance, a singer and guitarist, observed my plight and devised what sounded like the perfect scheme: wear the right cologne, go to the right bar, and meet someone. She assured me that with the ultimate European aftershave, I would have luck in Wilmington's classiest hangout for young professionals. I dutifully set out to meet the woman of my dreams.

I read the "Appropriate Dress Required" sign upon entering Baker's Tavern north of Wilmington and hoped my white Oxford shirt and jeans would do. Sitting down at the bar next to the only woman in the room, I ordered mineral water. I imagined that had piqued her curiosity, because almost right away she turned to me with a friendly smile and asked, "So, what do you do?" I allowed myself to believe that maybe she, too, had come hoping to meet a mate.

Again I fell back on honesty, my only strong suit. "Actually, I'm living with my father right now. I had a car accident a while back. I don't really do much of anything."

She looked at me as if waiting for me to say more.

I felt a little seasick as the seconds ticked by. Finally, a bit of Tatiana's advice occurred to me: get people to talk about themselves. "How about you?"

"I'm in sales." More silence.

"Oh," I said. What was "sales"? My awareness of the business world had always been sketchy. I had never picked up anyone in a bar before, and besides wearing the right cologne and going to the right place, I was out of my depth.

"Nice to meet you," she said, and got up to leave.

"Nice to meet you, too," I said. I stayed to finish my mineral water.

* * *

Next I looked up the "Quaker girl" who had opened my eyes to the necessity of being accepted for who and what I was. Surely she wouldn't discriminate against me or find me boorish. I remembered the closeness I had felt with the whole group at the retreat. We were already attracted to each other.

It sounded like a great idea, but it turned out that she had her own issues. If two people are going to work out together, somebody has to be stable at any particular moment, and back then I couldn't count on myself to be steady. And if I couldn't, she couldn't. Unfortunately, that went both ways.

Painfully needing female company, I then tried dating a young woman who lived in a convent. I knew that she was not a nun despite her living situation, but my awareness of her purity precluded some physical advances, and as a recently married man I had come to have expectations about my relationships with women.

Besides the need to respect her virtue, practical considerations entered the mix: in order for our relationship to work out, I would have to follow her home to the Netherlands and learn Dutch. I knew I was capable of a lot after my experience with Tatiana, but this time, to my surprise, the woman herself called off our courtship. "Can't read the handwriting on the wall?" I asked myself miserably, recalling the title of my high school op-ed article about people who are out of touch with reality.

I began to wonder if there was any way for a brain-injured, young manic depressive like me to ever find happiness.

Desperate, in the spring of 1997, I called my college sweetheart and asked to visit. Maybe because I had parted with her on such endearingly honest terms ten years earlier—in fact, when I had just fallen in love with Angela—

she took pity on me and invited me to spend some time in Washington, DC. She was not yet married.

"So, you only asked for a divorce because you wanted the freedom to look for someone new?" she said as we strolled through a park. Somehow, in spite of our breakup, we could still talk about intimate matters with each other, sort of like best friends.

"Yeah, that's right," I said. I later found out, to my complete surprise, that she herself was in a largely unsatisfactory relationship and would, following suit, drop her boyfriend and find someone else to marry.

CHAPTER 57

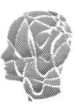

How to Make a Good Impression

It was already summer. In my early morning slumber, I dreamed that the made-in-China Valentine's teddy bear my father had given me was running on low batteries. Nevertheless, my dream self surreptitiously squeezed its pink "I Love You" heart to hear its fading song: "You are my sunshine . . ." I looked up to see my father watching me, smiling tenderly. Embarrassed, I shook myself awake, only to find it had been a dream, and I dozed until my alarm clock rudely beeped.

The morning sun was pouring in and "7:15" glowed red on the clock face. I pressed the snooze button. Pink pill bottles lay scattered on the floor. Peering at their labels, I shook out a lithium capsule, swallowed it whole with my saliva, then conked out for another ten minutes.

I hurried through my morning routine of showering, shaving, and walking downtown to the mayor's office. I walked home again around noon and then visited a neighborhood acquaintance. I lay exhausted from my three-hour day on his couch.

"Hey, Tom," he said, "I hear there's a party tonight in Arden." At the words "party" and "Arden," my ears pricked up. My friend had briefly lived there. "The woman who's throwing the party heads up the Delaware Literary Guild."

He knew I had recently been giving online dating a try, signing up for "Single Book Lovers," and that I was longing to meet a compatible woman. Arden had formerly been an artist's colony and was now a privileged counterculture community north of Wilmington, an even more likely venue than Single Book Lovers for encountering an intelligent partner.

My heart started beating in a familiar way, the way it did when I was most aware of being alive and knew I had something worthwhile to offer. I knew that I was meant to go and meet someone.

"You want to come along?" I asked.

"Nah. Say hello for me." I was already rushing out.

My mother's training kicked in: shave before appearing in public. I explained to the hostess that I had crashed her party and then made a beeline for the nearest single woman. She was attractive, petite, and older than me, wearing rhinestone sunglasses.

"So, where do you fit in?" she asked hopefully, ignoring the razor nicks on my face.

"Actually, I don't fit in anywhere," I began, again falling back on bald honesty. "I had a car accident several years ago. Brain damage. See?" I pointed to the left lens of my glasses, where an ingenious optometrist had dabbed clear nail polish to block the vision of that eye, which saw two images.

Of course she couldn't see my brain damage, any more than I could see hers, but I turned out to be the first person she'd met in the thirty years since her own injury who had also experienced brain trauma and not only felt free to mention it, but used it as a come-on.

"What's that?" she frowned, squinting. "Looks like nail polish."

In the 1960s, at the time of her concussion, she had been told never to mention her disability to anyone. She had taken this to heart so deeply that she didn't even mention it to herself. To her, my manner seemed bravely outspoken, not silly.

"I'm working on getting over my injury," I continued, trying to win her attention with my latest attempt at self-improvement, homeopathy.

"My mother always told me not to tell people," she confided. "She said people would discriminate. Aren't you afraid of that?"

"Soon I'll be so much better that it won't matter," I said.

She glossed over my grandiosity. "I guess attitudes have changed over the last thirty years." A pause. "Do you really think there's a cure? I don't see how there could be." She was obviously weighing the possibilities. "Well, if it works for you . . ."

Little did I know how much I had in common with this unusual woman I met because I followed my heart to a party.

I decided to lay all my cards on the table. "What would you say if I asked you out on a date?"

She looked up at me and smiled, glanced down for a second, then looked back into my eyes. "I guess I'd say yes. Have you ever been to Haverford's arboretum?"

"Haverford? I went to Haverford."

At this, I knew our match was made in heaven. We agreed to meet the following evening for a walk around the college's circuit trail.

CHAPTER 58

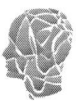

Finding Home

Joan, the woman I met at the party, took the broad view that there was at least something interesting about everything, including me. Damage to her temporal lobes, caused by her accident, gave her seizures that affected her emotions and sense of time. It also made her distractible, a problem complicated by her appreciation of what she perceived to be an endlessly fascinating world.

Having trained at nearby Longwood Gardens, she knew the botanical names for most plants. As we walked the trail, she stopped dead in her tracks, then leaned back and pointed. "Oh look, *Quercus acutissima*! Easy to identify in July. Fine example." She stepped off the path for a different view of the tree. I stood admiring her instead.

"You just don't see that very often around here." She looked up at me seriously.

Unable to keep track of much besides my own balance while walking on the rough trail, I tried to appear interested, wondering how the evening was going to end.

"Would you like to come back to my place for some tea?" she asked, surely reading my mind. "I don't live far." I followed her home, she in her sporty white hatchback, I in my old red Chevette, along roads already familiar to me from biking in my college days.

Her house stood in a row of tidy 1920s bungalows, each with a small lawn, facing another row of similar houses across a narrow street: an old-fashioned tight-knit suburban neighborhood, full of dogs, cats, mothers, and baby strollers. Children shrieked happily in a nearby schoolyard. A tree bloomed luxuriously in her front yard, red flowers spilled out of window boxes, and glass vases of all colors, beautifully backlit, shone on shelves in her porch windows.

I was drawn in by the relaxed and cozy atmosphere, and even more by her domesticity.

She unlocked the front door and let me in, saying, "I'm sorry, all I have is herbal tea." But I had forgotten about the tea. I stood in the living room in front of her fireplace, made out of large blackened stones, facing a sage-colored suede couch, and exclaimed involuntarily, "Oh Joan, I'd love to live here!"

She gasped quietly, then turned to me and smiled. "Well . . . maybe we could arrange that." I had already flopped down on the couch.

The following Monday, while I was away, she called her ex, whom she had continued to see every day for the previous year despite having made him move out. She wanted to call off their relationship for good. "I've met the man," she explained, "that I'm going to spend my life with."

I confess I was taken aback when she confided her rash decision to me. At the time, the only thing I could think to say was, "I'm so glad you're in touch with your feelings," hardly a declaration of undying love to match hers. I even told her that I doubted I could have feelings for anyone that were as deep as those I still had for Tatiana. She was glad for me that I had been so deeply in love.

I moved in at the end of the week, bringing with me only pill bottles and shoes, one set of clothes, and the white linen pants I wore to work. A few days later, I brought over a pair of jeans and two more shirts. What else could I possibly need?

Two weeks after that, I quit my job at the mayor's office in order to take up life full time with my new love.

Autumn is hard on many manic depressives, and that fall was no different for me. One evening while reading to Joan in her bathtub, I began to have the familiar swimming sensation in my head that accompanied loss of touch with reality. "Should I tell her how I feel?" I thought. I remembered Tatiana's panicked reaction and thought better of it, but then I only felt worse, alone in my misery.

"Joan," I finally mustered, looking up from the book.

"What is it, Tom?" I had been reading *The Arabian Nights*, and she had been enjoying the story.

I looked at her, wide eyed and scared. "I think I'm going crazy again." I had no idea how she would react.

She sat up in the tub and looked at me sweetly. Then she began to sing the song "Rag Doll" in a good imitation of Frankie Valli, substituting "Tom" for the word "Doll".

I let myself relax.

She kept singing: ". . . I love you just the way you are . . ."

Joan has a remarkable memory for lyrics and a great voice. This would not be the last time that she pulled the right song out of a hat at the appropriate moment. I realized that I had moved in with a person more accepting of me than I could ever have imagined.

"We can call my doctor. I'm sure he can straighten things out without having to put you in the hospital. His specialty is tough patients, but he hates institutions. Somehow he manages to get people stable at home." A trip to the hospital was my worst nightmare, and Joan's confidence, so unlike Tatiana's fear, put me at ease.

Her psychiatrist was, in fact, a wizard. Soon I left Dr. Spalding to be in his care. It turned out that, unlike previous doctors, he placed a big enough priority on my quality of life that he refused to keep me sedated. Lucky for me!

He had an extensive knowledge of neurology and experimented with combinations of medications. Soon I was able to handle minor household chores—meal preparation, shopping, laundry, dishes. I could even walk to the local library after I cleaned the bathroom.

The more alert I became, the more I was able to follow my father's example, not only by cooking but by searching beyond what MDs had to offer. I felt an ever-increasing desire to overcome my disability through alternative medicine.

* * *

Joan and I spent one of our first Sundays together attending a local Friends meeting, one that I had enjoyed visiting when I was a student. Just being in that setting helped to restore my identity. Besides resurrecting my Quaker roots, the place held a particular attraction for me because, although I had been devastated during recent years, my losses had only served to deepen my spiritual awareness. Staring at ceilings for so long had brought out in me a sort of monasticism. I had little else to do but reflect. She, on the other hand, had been meditating for twenty-five years and was quickly lost in worship.

The Quaker meeting caught us up in its bustle, and we soon were inspired to take on what seemed like enormous amounts of responsibility. This really meant that I volunteered and Joan did most of the work, something she enjoyed, even when it was largely clerical. I had little use for boring activities, but, true to form, she found something interesting in everything I volunteered us for. The meeting also served as a link to the alternative medical community in the Philadelphia area.

As always, I was constantly looking for new ways to heal. By driving one older member of the meeting to her weekly appointments, I met her psychiatrist, an eighty-some-year-old Reichian osteopath who antedated the rise of "Big Pharma." Reich, my friend explained, unlike Freud, worked on the premise that mental health could be brought about by freeing up the movement of energy in the body. That had a familiar "mind-body" sound to it that I liked.

As I waited in the psychiatrist's lobby, originally the living room of his Pine Street house, a huge blue-jacketed portrait of Reich himself stared down at me from the wall. I found out that the portrait, as well as perhaps eight original watercolors, were all the work of the doctor himself. I leafed through a book he had recently written, which lay on a nearby table, and my eye alit on his words: "From the perspective of psychiatric orgone therapy (orgone is the name Reich gave to the energy which moves us), we are descending into a Dark Ages in the practice of psychiatry." This was my kind of shrink.

While he very much preferred that his patients remain unmedicated if at all possible, he recognized the importance of keeping me on lithium and the antipsychotic. He still did daily chin-ups, undeterred by the passing of years; encouraged vacations for stress relief and mental health; and prescribed exercise to encourage the body to sleep. When my own dad got fed up with my endless and seemingly groundless optimism—he eventually even stopped answering my phone calls—I still found a father figure in the Reichian.

Joan, unlike Tatiana, was a tireless and practical homemaker. When not puttering in her overflowing garden, which she would often tend throughout the afternoon and into moonlight, she would mend clothing or repair things in her basement. She was the kind of warm and down-to-earth woman I had never had in my mother.

Our wedding took place in our meetinghouse nearby, not at my father's place in Wilmington. The service was simple—Quakers feel no need for clergy—followed by an informal reception.

"I never thought he would find love again," my father said during the ceremony, tears in his eyes, "I'm so happy he has found someone who sees him for what he is and loves him."

Maybe the distance from my father's house convinced Ingeborg not to boycott this ceremony. Or maybe she wanted to pay respects to Joan's family, who did not have far to come, unlike the parents of my previous bride. Ingeborg made a hasty exit, though, well before the photographer could catch her anywhere near my father.

CHAPTER 59

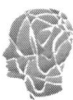

A Second Chance

Several years into our marriage, in early 2004, I awoke with a start from a nightmare. Joan was sleeping soundly beside me. In the dream, my parents were walking down a country road in Germany. He was telling her how a mutual friend had died, a gifted composer. "Shot in the head nine times in a Russian prison camp," he said. My mother clapped her hands to her cheeks and wailed, running away down the road. Nine times!

I only told Joan about it later that day while we were working out at the YMCA. The powerful dream left me feeling unusually confused and weak, very unlike myself.

"Joan," I said, coming over to sit by her exercise bicycle, "I had a nightmare this morning." She slowed down and drifted to a stop. "Of course I've always known that I had a brain injury, but now I really know it. I can feel it. 'Shot in the head nine times.' The old me died—I saw my parents grieving. My mother was horrified."

Joan didn't miss a beat. She slid off the bike and came over to take my hand. "Maybe until now you weren't ready to feel this way, Tom. Dreams only present things to you when you're ready. Maybe it's time for you to grieve, too."

Until that day, I had been carefully planning my return to Columbia in my prior field, political science. Suddenly I realized how incapable I was of even reading signs on the walls of the gym. How absurd it was to think I could handle graduate study.

Still shaken, that Sunday I confided my dream to a fellow Quaker during coffee hour. I did not know at the time that he was a psychiatrist. His first question was, "Do you have a social worker?"

I was overcome by even more doubt. "No," I said, "I only have Joan."

* * *

Later that spring, the elderly woman who had introduced me to the Reichian psychiatrist had to move out of her house to a retirement home. The entire Quaker community helped her go through her packratted possessions. For our part, Joan and I visited her frequently in the new facility. She and her son were estranged, and I felt a special affinity for her. Although alone, she was in remarkably good spirits on many of our visits.

One visit, though, she was particularly morose. "What happened, Cynthia?" I asked as we sat together at a lunch table on her locked ward.

"They washed my orgone blanket. They swiped it while I was doing therapy."

Cynthia had always been given to somewhat off-the-wall remarks, and I thought this was another one. "What's wrong with that, Cynthia? Even if it wasn't that dirty, won't it be cleaner now?"

Cynthia put her head in her hands and cried.

"No, you don't understand," she said eventually, looking up at us with teary eyes. "It has steel wool in it. That's what makes it worth having. Now it's ruined—the water rusted it." The loss of Cynthia's orgone blanket initiated her real decline in the nursing facility.

In a message to my mother later, I mentioned the orgone blanket incident in connection with a book I was sending her. Because of double vision, I hadn't been able to read the book myself, but after Joan summarized it for me I thought it would help Ingeborg understand me better. I got an e-mail back the next day, its text highlighted in color: "I had *no idea* you would ever visit an *old woman* in the hospital. *You never cease to surprise me.*" The blue letters glowed from my screen.

I was surprised at her response. Actually, maybe she was talking about the me she used to know. I had just been doing what came naturally these days.

Ingeborg committed suicide soon after, carrying out the wish she had stated repeatedly for the previous twenty-five years.

CHAPTER 60

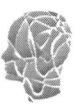

Thank God I Married a Saint

Before she moved out of her home, Cynthia had also introduced me to her acupuncturist. He had cured himself of a brain injury, placing acupuncture needles into his head by looking in a mirror. He had learned from an Indian master in California in the 1970s and had treated Cynthia for years. He specialized in accident injuries and other tough cases. He had a welcome streak of generosity. Like my shaman friend in Wilmington, he would often treat me for free, allowing me to pay only when my guilty conscience caught up with me.

The same year, a friend invited us to spend two weeks in a summer cabin at the seaside in Maine. I prepared for the trip less carefully than I had for the summer in Russia: only one set of pills, which I kept in the car's glove compartment. After all, a pharmacy would be nearby.

On the drive up we stopped near Boston to spend the night with Friends.

"So what do you do?" our host asked, once we had settled in and taken our places at the dinner table.

Rather than go into a long account, I ventured, "I'm writing a book about my life." Joan nodded encouragingly.

Our friends looked at each other knowingly. "Whatever you do, don't keep your writing on a computer in a closed car. This summer's going to be a hot one. We know someone who lost her whole book that way." Oh, right… the heat! I wondered if I should rescue my meds before they got cooked in the glove compartment, but didn't follow up. In retrospect, I wish I had.

* * *

A week later, the cabin had turned into a nightmare. My pills had lost their potency and I was in the grips of white-hot mania. I had volunteered to give the cabin its seasonal housecleaning in return for free utilities but was leaving all the cleaning to Joan. It irritated me that she was working so diligently and seemed oblivious of me.

"Joan, can't you knock off the cleaning? I need the keys to your car. I want to sell the stock I just bought. I need to send hard copy right away."

She looked up from her scrub brush.

"Joan, I just have this gut feeling. You know how good I am with my intuition."

"Hey, Tom, this is the third desperate transaction you've put through since this time yesterday. Each one has meant an hour-and-a-half round trip. That's a lot of driving for someone on vacation."

"Joan, are our finances important to you, or just to me?"

"This is beginning to make me uncomfortable, Tom. Maybe we should sleep on it." She looked up at me and smiled appealingly, raising her eyebrows. Her body language was saying, "Hey, be reasonable."

Something in me snapped. "Goddamn it, Joan! Just give me the f*cking keys!" I crashed my fist on the nearby table. As she stared at me, I registered the shock in her eyes but not her glazed-over retreat into herself. I heard her breathe out, trying to exhale fully. With her next breath she stood, not even seeming to notice she was leaving the scrub brush on the floor where I might trip over it. She started for the door, and by the time her feet left the porch, she was running. Soon she disappeared in the direction of the shore. In the distance I heard a wild roar echoing across the water, but it didn't occur to me to worry for her.

Almost immediately I saw our host emerge from his cabin and join her on the beach. I was gathering my things to leave when I heard the screen door open. She and our friend, a psychology professor, had been chatting. By now he was near enough to catch my eye.

"Did anyone hear a bear?" he asked innocently. His cabin, a stone's throw from our own, faces the same shore. "You have to be careful this time of year."

Joan turned back to him. "Come on. I just told you that was me. I had some bad energy I had to get out." No mention of her husband. Joan is a masterful diplomat, one of the many things I love about her.

Our friend glanced at me, then back at Joan. "Well, that's a relief. That's a healthy way to deal with emotions. Bears can be dangerous."

When we returned from Maine, Joan wasted no time kicking me out, saying she wished she had driven home alone and left me there way before the two-week trip was over. I spent the first night out of the house with Carter, my Haverford cycling friend. He and his wife now lived nearby.

Carter was not up for extended hospitality, so for the second night I called my father. "Aren't you and Joan getting along?" he asked over the phone. I could hear his concern.

"We just need a little time apart. It'll only be one night," I said, hoping we could somehow patch it up in a day.

"Tom, I'm getting old. Of course you can come, but I won't be living here much longer. I'm moving into a retirement community soon and won't have an extra bed."

"Thanks, Dad."

I'm not sure why, but Joan accepted me back the following day. Maybe she figured that the depleted drugs were to blame for my problems, or that I would improve with time. Getting kicked out became a touchstone for me: from then on, I would never again let myself get that far out of control.

CHAPTER 61

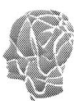

Climbing Mount Sinai

After treating me for several years, Cynthia's acupuncturist recommended that I get comprehensive brain injury testing. He knew that I had dropped out of rehabilitation many years before, but he needed to establish a baseline for his treatment. I dutifully made an appointment at nearby Bryn Mawr Rehabilitation.

At the time, my memory was still porous, my math skills were terrible, and my brain's ability to initiate tasks had not yet returned. This time, instead of just sweating as I had at my research job interview a few years earlier, I threw up in a trash can during the test. "Shall we continue now?" asked my interviewer, nonplussed. Thoroughly demoralized, I pushed on, ending up with an IQ of just over 100.

The acupuncturist was angry that I had been treated so poorly, and that I'd had to pay for the privilege, too. Though the test had provided important information, it had come at the cost of my morale. "I'll get retested at a different facility," I thought.

I applied to the state's Office of Vocational Rehabilitation to get the funding needed for evaluation at MossRehab, the much-respected hospital from which I had been transferred as a disruptive maniac almost a decade before.

At Moss, now operating as an outpatient, I demonstrated my functional ability by performing a series of tasks and did considerably better than when I had undergone strictly cognitive tests. Could I balance a checkbook? Could I assemble a widget? Of course I could, not that I ever did in real life.

While at Moss, I mentioned that I was writing a book. "The best book so far on brain injury is by Claudia Osborn," one of the therapists told me. Osborn was a Michigan doctor who had gotten hit by a car while bicycling and was rehabilitated at NYU's Rusk Rehabilitation Institute in New York City. When I got home, I ordered her book through the library and plowed my way through her story, double vision and all.

Dr. Osborn's case bore some resemblance to mine: a terrible accident involving a promising young person. But she, I read, had received comprehensive rehabilitation at one of the best facilities in the country, whereas I had dropped out of rehabilitation for personal reasons. Her story was in the back of my mind when I next ran across reference to a famous New York rehab and research facility.

In late 2008, I got a job writing for an online newspaper, *The Examiner*. My beat was "Philadelphia Health." It gave me the opportunity to extemporize in print on my favorite topic, alternative medicine. Joan read over my articles before I submitted them. I was paid a pittance, but I took the job seriously, since it was building a portfolio of recent journalistic work.

One article I had planned was going to address brain injury and alternative medicine. I came across Mount Sinai on the Web, and thought that perhaps I could share some wisdom with them about how to treat brain injury. When I found myself talking with their admissions director on the phone, though, I realized that Mount Sinai could do more for me than I could for them.

"We are conducting a pilot study on problem solving for people with brain injuries of long standing," she said. "It wouldn't cost you anything. You would have to come up for testing to see if you qualify."

"Could I commute from Philadelphia?"

"You'd have to stay in New York City for three nights a week, but we have had commuters before."

I did some quick calculations in my head: I had about three good friends in and around New York City. If I divided my time among them, chances were that I could swing it. "I'll be there," I said, pleased at a coincidence that was paving my way effortlessly, like old times. It was meant to happen! Just then, though, I broke my ankle on a trip to see my father. Not to be deterred, I packed off to New York in an orthopedic boot of impressive dimensions.

***

"What's your biggest remaining deficit from the accident?" the intake coordinator asked me in her office in Mount Sinai's elaborate basement complex on East 98th Street.

"I can't read a book," I said. "I used to be a graduate student, and now I can't read," My voice broke with emotion.

"We are going to send you back to Columbia!" my interviewer declared triumphantly. From what I had read about Mount Sinai, if anyone could do it, they could.

When I emerged from her office, I sat down next to a young man, evidently another traumatic brain injury (TBI) survivor. Both of us watched, surprised, as a psychologist limped by in front of us wearing a huge black ankle boot reminiscent of mine. "One of the country's premier foot injury centers," he smiled, gesturing at my own leg.

I spent the following twelve weeks in the spring of 2009 commuting on the rails between Philadelphia and New York City, getting up before the crack of dawn every Tuesday morning in order to arrive before classes started. Hope, my Columbia friend from my days with Tatiana, offered me gracious hospitality, as did two other friends. By rotating hosts and shuffling weeks here and there, I never had to stay in a hotel.

Rehabilitation focused mainly on problem solving. I joined a small group of other TBI survivors for classes led by talented young PhD psychologists in Mount Sinai's stuffy basement classrooms. We learned to define problems, brainstorm on solutions, and then implement them. I felt empowered: I had never been taken so seriously since my accident, especially at a brain injury rehab facility, and told my group so.

"They sure took your money seriously in Philadelphia, though," one group member joked.

At the end of my rehabilitation, I was confident enough to call Columbia and ask to be reenrolled.

* * *

In 2010, Joan and I attended a zoning meeting in a local elementary school auditorium. An ambitious local entrepreneur was challenging a standing township ordinance, claiming it violated his right to free speech by keeping him from erecting huge billboards along neighborhood thoroughfares. Fearing the loss of her property's value, not to mention the addition of an eyesore, Joan had decided to fight.

She attended the next zoning board hearing dressed as a proper Main Line matron, a far cry from her usual gardening outfit, and even coiffed herself for the occasion. She deliberately arrived half an hour early to mingle and scope out the opposition.

"So, how do you feel about these billboards?" she asked casually as she sat down behind an equally well-dressed man. He was the only other person in the room.

"Actually, I'm just here on official business," he said. "How about you?"

"I think they're dangerous. After all, the whole point of them is to attract your attention." The man was listening seriously, so she continued. "I've been distracted by billboards badly enough that I've almost caused accidents. Me! And I was driving by myself, nobody else talking in the other seats to confuse me, no phone . . . We'd have a huge uptick in accidents in our township. Scares me!"

"You'd be surprised that the statistics don't bear you out," said the man, who turned out to be the expert witness for the billboard entrepreneur's lawyer.

"That's hard to believe!"

"Think what you like." He smiled, then added, "Just don't tell the zoning board what you told me. I don't need anyone drawing my credibility into question."

"Oh? So nice talking to you, Mister . . . what's your name? I'm so glad we met." She offered her hand and the most polite of Main Line smiles.

Joan skipped into our home at 10 p.m. "Can you believe the nerve of that guy?" she called. "Willing to ruin our neighborhood just to make some money? I think he's the stooge of the billboard interests!" I got up from my seat at our computer and ran to meet her.

"What's up?"

"He brought on an expert witness from a state agency saying that billboards cause absolutely no traffic hazard, even those ones that light up and change pictures every couple of seconds! Those guys will say anything. I don't know, apparently he represents the highway commission. Hard to argue with that."

"Did he say anything else?"

"Yeah, he told me for God's sake not to mention in front of the zoning board how easily drivers get distracted."

Wheels started turning in my mind. Sure, I'd been disabled for over ten years. Maybe now was the time to put my condition to some positive use. Maybe I was not just hit by a truck, but by a distracted truck driver. Sure, he had been distracted by the snow. But it could just as well have been . . . a billboard!

"Joan, I've got it! You've done it!"

"What? What have I done?"

"You've ended billboards in our township!"

I quickly filed a petition to speak at the next hearing and spent hours during the next few days keying search after search into the Google box. Finally I hit on it: a recent international study documenting that billboards were unsafe. Plenty of statistics and charts. At the next hearing, yes, I still spoke with a lisp. And my voice was trembling with emotion. My gait was still broken as I made my way to the front of the boardroom. But that only served to strengthen my case, because I was going to appear in public not as an Ivy League graduate, but rather as a disabled resident who would be speaking from personal experience in order to make the case even more persuasive.

- The End -

EPILOGUE

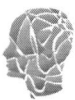

Huge billboards never appeared on any of our township's roads. I eventually returned to Columbia University's Harriman Institute as a graduate student, this time not to study political science, but to write about alternative medicine for brain injury.

On a summer visit to Germany, Joan and I were hosted for several nights by my Düsseldorf love, now slim and working as a diplomat. She is happily married with three children.

I continue my friendship with Tatiana, who refers to Joan as "awesome." Joan handles Tatiana's finances here in the US so that she can maintain her dual citizenship.

A map of my brain's signals done using the low-energy neurofeedback system (LENS) in 2011 showed that I still had considerable deficits. Two years later, after various alternative therapies, including LENS, a similar evaluation charted funtioning approaching optimal.

As far as bipolar illness goes, I eventually found an orthomolecular physician who is transitioning me to vitamins and supplements to control my moods, thus obviating the need for medication.

CHRONOLOGY

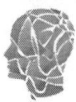

July 1988 - Study German in Düsseldorf

August 1988 - Disowned by mother

September 1988 - Enter Moscow's Pushkin Institute to study Russian

October 1988 - Meet Tatiana

January 1989 - Enter Plekhanov Institute in Moscow to study Russian

June 1989 - First cycling tour by Russians through the US

July 1989 - First American cycling tour through the Soviet Union

September 1989 - Enter Columbia University in New York

December 1989 - Marry Tatiana

July 1990 - Study German in Bavaria

July 1991 - Committed to Soviet mental hospital; given ECT

August 1991- Moscow mayor Boris Yeltsin's coup

August 1991- Rescued by father and flown back to US

August 1991 - Committed to Wilmington (Delaware) mental hospital

January 1992 - Return to Columbia

September 1992 - Move to Bryn Mawr (Pennsylvania) with Tatiana

February 1993 - Car T-boned by eighteen-wheeler

March 1993 - Committed to Einstein Hospital's psychiatric ward

May 1993 - Committed to Jefferson Hospital's psychiatric ward

June 1993 - Check out of brain injury rehabilitation

July 1993 - Given acupuncture and Chinese herbs

September 1993 - Take Tibetan pills

October 1993 - Russian president Yeltsin shells his parliament building

November 1993 - Volunteer for mayor's office in Wilmington

February 1995 - Committed to Wilmington's psychiatric facility

August 1995 - Tatiana suffers a nervous breakdown and returns home

September 1996 - Divorce Tatiana

July 1997 - Meet Joan

December 1999 - Marry Joan

For more information about an
Annual Conference on Alternative Medicine for TBI
contact
Thomas E. Hartmann
hartmann.t.e@gmail.com
www.carnelianhealing.org